The Fasting Revolution

Revolutionize Your Body's Rhythms Through Intermittent Fasting

David Alexander

D1526744

Preface

In the ever-evolving landscape of health and wellness, a groundbreaking movement is taking shape, challenging the traditional notions of nourishment and wellbeing. "The Fasting Revolution: Revolutionize Your Body's Rhythms Through Intermittent Fasting" emerges as a pivotal work in this transformative journey. This book is not merely a guide; it is a manifesto that calls upon the reader to embark on a journey of self-discovery and radical change.

As you navigate through these pages, prepare to encounter a narrative that intertwines the intricate science of intermittent fasting with personal anecdotes and historical perspectives. Alexander's writing style is characterized by a unique blend of perplexity and burstiness, offering a reading experience that is as unpredictable as it is enlightening. The text oscillates between deeply technical explanations and sudden leaps into broader philosophical realms, mirroring the very nature of intermittent fasting. This practice defies linear understanding and requires an embrace of complexity.

"The Fasting Revolution" does not merely present fasting as a dietary choice; it repositions it as a radical alteration of life rhythms. Alexander proposes that by altering our eating patterns, we are not just changing our diet; we are reprogramming our biological clocks, reshaping our physiological narratives, and redefining our relationship with food. The book delves into the historical and cultural significance of fasting, tracing its roots and evolution, thereby providing a rich contextual background against which the modern practice is contrasted.

However, this book is not an echo chamber of existing fasting literature. Alexander challenges established beliefs, questions the status quo, and offers fresh perspectives on what it means to fast. His approach is not prescriptive but exploratory, encouraging readers to question, experiment, and find a path that resonates with their bodies and lifestyles.

In essence, "ThIn the ever-evolving landscape of health and wellness, a groundbreaking movement is taking shape, challenging the traditional notions of nourishment and wellbeing. "The Fasting Revolution: Revolutionize Your Body's Rhythms Through Intermittent Fasting" by David Alexander emerges as a pivotal work in this transformative journey. This book is not merely a guide; it is a manifesto that calls upon the reader to embark on a journey of self-discovery and radical change.

As you navigate through these pages, prepare to encounter a narrative that intertwines the intricate science of intermittent fasting with personal anecdotes and historical perspectives. Alexander's writing style is characterized by a unique blend of perplexity and burstiness, offering a reading experience that is as unpredictable as it is enlightening. The text oscillates between deeply technical explanations and sudden leaps into broader philosophical realms, mirroring the very nature of intermittent fasting – a practice that defies linear understanding and requires an embrace of complexity.

"The Fasting Revolution" does not merely present fasting as a dietary choice; it repositions it as a radical alteration of life rhythms. Alexander proposes that by altering our eating patterns, we are not just changing our diet; we are reprogramming our biological clocks, reshaping our physiological narratives, and redefining our relationship with food. The book delves into the historical and cultural significance of fasting, tracing its roots and evolution, thereby providing a rich contextual background against which the modern practice is contrasted.

However, this book is not an echo chamber of existing fasting literature. Alexander challenges established beliefs, questions the status quo, and offers fresh perspectives on what it means to fast. His approach is not prescriptive but exploratory, encouraging readers to question, experiment, and find a path that resonates with their individual bodies and lifestyles.

In essence, "The Fasting Revolution" is an invitation to a journey that is as much about self-exploration as it is about health. It's an adventurous foray into the unknown territories of human metabolism and psychology. As you turn each page, expect to be confronted with questions that defy easy answers and be prepared to engage with concepts that may fundamentally alter your understanding of nutrition and health.

The Fasting Revolution" is an invitation to a journey that is as much about self-exploration as it is about health. It's an adventurous foray into the unknown territories of human metabolism and psychology. As you turn each page, expect to be confronted with questions that defy easy answers, and be prepared to engage with concepts that may fundamentally alter your understanding of nutrition and health.

Welcome to the revolution. Welcome to a new rhythm of life.

David Alexander

Contents

Introduction   1

1. The Weight Loss Conundrum   5

2. Intermittent Fasting   13

3. The Health Benefits Beyond the Scale   23

4. Finding Your Fasting Rhythm   33

5. The Psychology of Fasting   45

6. Nutritional Strategies for Effective Fasting   55

7. Fasting and Exercise   63

8. Hormonal Harmony and Fasting   71

9. Fasting for Women   81

10. Managing Social and Lifestyle Factors   91

11. Advanced Fasting Protocols   99

12. Common Questions and Troubleshooting   107

Conclusion   115

Appendix A   119

Appendix B   123

Introduction

Unveiling the Secret of Sustainable Weight Loss

We all desire that magical solution, the one that effortlessly sheds unwanted pounds and brings us vibrant health. However, experience has taught us that sustainable weight loss cannot be found in a bottle. It stems from understanding our body's inner workings and achieving a balance that goes beyond just shedding weight; it's about embracing a healthier, happier life.

Now, envision a world where you are no longer trapped in the cycle of yo-yo dieting. Imagine bidding farewell to calorie counting, food deprivation, and the guilt associated with any dietary slip-ups. This isn't a mere fantasy; it is the reality awaiting you when you embrace intermittent fasting.

But don't be alarmed by the term "fasting." We are not referring to extreme fasting methods where you survive on nothing but lemon water for days on end. Instead, we are talking about a structured and scientifically supported approach to eating (or not eating) that rejuvenates your metabolism, frees your mind from constant food thoughts, and leads to sustainable weight loss.

1

Traditional diets often set us up for disappointment. They tend to focus more on external solutions for what is primarily an internal issue. It's not just about the number of calories in our food, but rather how our bodies react to those calories. This is the major flaw in many weight loss strategies—they fail to address the underlying reasons why our bodies hold onto fat like a lifebuoy.

Enter intermittent fasting, a secret weapon of sorts. This approach isn't solely about drastically cutting calories; it's more about when you eat. By reorganizing the timing of our meals, we can trigger significant and positive transformations in our bodies that extend well beyond just the number on the weighing scale.

But why isn't this common knowledge? Why isn't everyone adopting this method? Well, there's a lot of misinformation out there—myths and misconceptions that present an incomplete picture of what fasting truly entails. Throughout these pages, we will dispel confusion and bring clarity and simplicity to the concept of intermittent fasting.

However, we have quite a journey ahead of us—one that will uncover the intricacies of your metabolism, shed light on the scientific basis behind fasting's effects, and explain why it may contradict everything you previously believed about dieting.

As we delve into the depths of genuine health through fasting, we will explore benefits that extend far beyond what shows up on your bathroom scale.

Let's explore the benefits of fasting, such as promoting longevity, reducing disease risk, and improving mental well being.

It's important to note that there isn't a one-size-fits-all approach. That's why we'll assist you in discovering your own fasting routine. Whether you prefer mornings or evenings, enjoy leisurely walks or intense workouts at the gym, we'll help you find a fasting schedule that seamlessly fits into your lifestyle.

Adjusting to a new eating pattern can be mentally challenging alongside the physical aspects. Therefore, we will equip you with strategies to reshape your mindset, overcome psychological obstacles, and establish a positive relationship with food as nourishment rather than an adversary.

By combining the principles of fasting with nutritional knowledge, we will ensure that when you do eat, the food on your plate supports and sustains your fasting efforts alongside incorporating exercise into this holistic plan tailored just for you.

Recognizing that everybody is unique and complex, we will also address specific concerns certain groups may have—such as women who navigate different hormonal landscapes during significant life stages like pregnancy or menopause.

Life, as we all know, doesn't exist in isolation. Navigating social commitments, finding work life balance, and staying on track even while traveling. These are all interconnected aspects that we'll help you manage. We will guide you on adapting without compromising your goals.

As you become more confident in your fasting routine, we will explore advanced protocols and delve into the fascinating process of autophagy. Where your body rejuvenates itself at a cellular level. Don't worry if this sounds complicated; we're here to simplify the science for you.

The pursuit of sustainable weight loss isn't about deprivation and strict rules; it's an exciting journey to uncover what your body can achieve when you pay attention to it and align with its natural rhythms. Are you ready to embark on this enlightening path towards sustainable well being? Let's begin this transformative exploration of lasting health together.

Chapter 1

The Weight Loss Conundrum

Why is it that despite the abundance of diet plans, fitness routines and weight loss advice available to us, many people still find themselves caught in an endless cycle of losing and gaining weight? One would assume that with all the information out there, shedding a few pounds would be a straightforward task. However, here's the catch: weight loss goes beyond simply eating less and exercising more. It involves comprehending the intricate interplay between metabolism, nutrition and physiology. In this section, let's explore the complexities of the common struggle with weight loss and begin to untangle the various factors that have ensnared countless individuals who prioritize their health.

Each year brings forth a new fad in diets that claim to be the ultimate solution for weight management. However, statistics paint a different picture by highlighting repeated disappointments and setbacks. It is hard to admit, but most diets fall short because they are rooted in outdated myths and misconceptions. Relying on quick fixes or restricting oneself to specific food groups is no longer effective as it fails to acknowledge our body's inherent wisdom. Nevertheless, traditional diet culture continues to endorse these approaches – perhaps it is time for a dietary revolution.

To truly grasp the essence of effective and sustainable weight loss, we must shift our perspective and recognize that it might be simpler than we imagine.

Let's be real: dieting can be appealing. We're attracted to the notion of becoming a slimmer and healthier version of ourselves. However, we often underestimate the emotional toll that strict and restrictive diets can take on us. Instead of nourishing our bodies, we find ourselves locked in a constant battle against them. So, let's put aside all the confusing diet beliefs and explore how intermittent fasting could revolutionize our approach. It's time to move beyond exhausting struggles with weight and embrace a more balanced lifestyle that aligns with our natural biology. But before we delve deeper into the specifics in upcoming sections, let's pause for a moment and reconsider our collective approach to dieting. Together, we can discover a way to break free from this perpetual enigma of weight loss once and for all.

Redefining Diet Culture

So, we've delved into the tangled web of conventional weight loss wisdom and seen just how convoluted it can get. Now, it's time to turn the tables and redefine the narratives that have long dictated our relationship with food and our bodies. Let's start peeling back the layers of diet culture, a beast that has touted a one-size-fits-all solution to what is undeniably a complex, multifaceted issue.

What exactly is diet culture? At its core, it's a belief system that values thinness, appearance, and shape above health and well-being. This approach demonizes certain ways of eating while glorifying others, often resulting in cycles of severe restriction followed by inevitable binges. It's this very paradigm that has led so many astray on their journeys toward sustainable health.

Why cling to a formula that so clearly isn't working for the masses? The truth is traditional diets tend to be result-oriented, fixated on immediate, often drastic outcomes. They're hinged on short-term deprivation instead of long-term lifestyle changes. We've been misled into equating health with the numbers on a scale, ignoring our body's fundamental needs for nourishment and satisfaction.

It's time for a monumental shift. Take intermittent fasting, for example—a practice that tears down the traditional scaffolding of 'dieting' by encouraging an eating pattern that aligns more naturally with our body's innate rhythms. This isn't about banning entire food groups or living on calorie deficits that leave you famished; it's about granting your body the time it needs to use what it has efficiently.

Redefining diet culture starts with embracing the idea that healthy living is not synonymous with constant restriction. It's recognizing that our bodies are diverse, with unique needs and responses to food. It's understanding that the quality of the food we consume is as crucial, if not more so, than the quantity.

So, how do we navigate this redefinition in practical terms? We can start by acknowledging the power of mindful eating—learning to listen to our hunger cues and eating not just for the sake of eating, but to fuel and satiate our bodies. It's also about finding balance, where movement and enjoyment of food go hand in hand, rather than viewing exercise as punishment for dietary choices.

By stepping away from the calorie-counting, meal-measuring mindset, we open ourselves up to a more intuitive way of living. And in doing so, we become more in tune with the natural signals our bodies send us. Intermittent fasting isn't a silver bullet, but it's a tool that can promote this attunement by simplifying our eating patterns and reducing the constant feedback loop of hunger and satiety signals that relentless snacking and frequent meals often create.

Another key to dismantling damaging diet culture is eliminating the shame and stigma associated with weight. It's essential to shift the focus from aesthetics to health, redefining success not as reaching a certain size but as building a lifestyle that leads to a sense of well-being and vitality.

Moreover, it's crucial to unlearn the notion that there are "good" and "bad" foods, and instead understand that context and moderation are what really matter. With intermittent fasting, when you eat, it becomes a lever to pull, adding flexibility and resilience to your diet rather than cultivating a punitive approach to certain foods.

In redefining diet culture, let's also challenge the hyperbolic language that often accompanies traditional dieting—words like 'cheat', 'sinful', and 'guilt-free'. Food is not a moral choice; it's a source of nourishment. Framing it within a moral context only adds to the emotional turmoil around eating and body image.

It's essential, too, to equip ourselves with knowledge. Understanding the biological mechanisms that underpin our eating habits can empower us to create more sustainable and effective approaches to healthy living. Intermittent fasting offers a glimpse into the sophistication of our body's natural processes, such as the cycle between fed and fasting states, and how they can be used to our advantage.

Tearing down the pillars of conventional diet culture isn't about abandoning the concept of health—it's about rebuilding it on terms that foster a more compassionate and sensible relationship with our bodies. We should no longer subject ourselves to regimens that breed discontent and disconnection from ourselves.

As we redefine diet culture, we find that the simplicity and liberation inherent in intermittent fasting can create a framework for a more sustainable lifestyle that dismisses the punitive restrictions of the past. This fresh perspective isn't just about losing weight—it's about gaining life, a richer, more fulfilling one that values health and happiness in equal measure.

Let's be clear—redefining diet culture doesn't imply that change is easy. It's a journey that demands introspection, patience, and often, unlearning ingrained patterns. But as we step away from the shadow of diet dogma, we step into the sunlight where food is not feared, where eating patterns sync with life's rhythms, and where health is holistically defined. Intermittent fasting offers a pathway out of the diet maze—it's up to us to take those steps toward a better, more balanced way of being.

Unpacking Common Dieting Myths

Let's break down some walls, shall we? Here we are, standing in the midst of a diet-culture debris field cluttered with myths that have long misled even the best of us. The idea behind weight loss sounds deceptively simple – eat less, move more. Yet, as many have found, simple doesn't necessarily mean easy or effective.

Myth number one that needs some serious debunking: "Eat a low-fat diet to lose fat." It's been a longstanding belief that fat on our plate translates directly to fat on our hips, but that's not entirely accurate. Our bodies require fats for essential processes, and what matters more is the type of fat we're eating. Healthy fats, like those found in avocados, fish, and nuts, can actually support weight loss by keeping us full and satisfied.

Falling in line next is the myth: "Calories in, calories out is all that matters." If losing weight were as simple as arithmetic, wouldn't we all be mathematicians with rock-solid abs? It's not merely the calories, but the quality of those calories and the timing of when you eat them that wield much greater significance. People may eat the same number of calories but experience vastly different outcomes.

And let's not forget the myth "Skipping meals leads to weight gain." While this can be true for some very specific dietary patterns, this assumption has terrified many from the thought of fasting, even intermittent fasting, which, spoiler alert, can actually be a proactive tool in weight management. The body is adaptable and can shift to burning stored fat for fuel.

We've all heard this one: "Eating small, frequent meals boosts your metabolism." Sounds plausible, right? However, the truth is that the 'metabolic boost' from eating more often is minimal at best. There's scant evidence supporting the idea that more meals lead to more weight loss; in fact, it could lead to more calorie consumption over the day.

Then there's the "Diet foods help you lose weight" myth. These products, often labeled as low-fat, fat-free, or sugar-free, can be deceptive. They frequently contain artificial sweeteners and other additives to compensate for reduced flavor. These substitutes can still spike insulin levels and potentially lead to more cravings and eventual weight gain.

The weight loss world is rife with the "You must exercise to lose weight" myth. Exercise is fundamentally good for our health, but its role in weight loss is often overstated. Depending on exercise alone without addressing dietary habits is like trying to bail out a boat with a sieve – hardly effective. It's about finding the right balance between diet and physical activity.

Now, take the myth that "Carbs are the enemy." This oversimplified idea ignores the fact that the human body needs carbohydrates for energy. It's the type of carbs – think whole grains versus refined sugars – that play a pivotal role in maintaining a healthy weight, not to mention overall health.

Let's also tackle the idea that "Weight loss is linear." If your journey doesn't resemble a sleek downhill slope, you're not alone. Weight fluctuates naturally, and plateaus are a normal part of the process. The body resists change; it's wired for survival, not for fitting into those jeans from high school.

"Healthy eating is all or nothing" is yet another myth. This black-and-white thinking has derailed many, as one slip-up can lead to feelings of failure and subsequent binge-eating. Sustainable eating habits allow for flexibility and forgiveness, embodying more of a balanced lifestyle than a rigorous diet.

And then there's this gem: "Supplements can replace dieting." If only it were so easy. Supplements might support a healthy diet, but they can't take the wheel. Solid nutrition comes from real, wholesome foods – and there's no magic pill that can replicate that.

The myth "Don't eat past 6 PM to lose weight" has become a modern dietary bedtime story. Our bodies don't suddenly stockpile fat after a specific hour. What's more important is the total caloric intake and output throughout the day, rather than the clock dictating your eating windows – a concept that intermittent fasting understands well.

Let's not overlook the "Detox diets cleanse your body for weight loss" myth. The body has an impressive detox system – the liver, kidneys, and intestines. While moderate detox diets can jumpstart a commitment to healthy eating, extensive detoxing is often unnecessary and ineffective for long-term weight loss.

Lastly, "To lose fat, avoid fats" is another misunderstanding that needs to go. The notion that all fats are bad is like saying all music is bad because you don't like a few genres. Our bodies need fat – it's a major energy source, and fats play a crucial role in hormone production, including hormones that regulate weight.

Exposing these myths is like turning on the lights at a masquerade ball. Suddenly, everything that once glistened suspiciously in the dark comes into stark relief. By casting off these chunky, ill-fitting myths, we embrace a more enlightened approach to weight loss. It's here, in this honest space, that something like intermittent fasting can step forward – not as another fad, but as a scientifically grounded method poised to revolutionize our relationship with food and our bodies.

Chapter 2

Intermittent Fasting

An Overview

As we turn the page from the tangled web of diet myths and misconceptions, let's zoom in on a concept that's been a game-changer for many: intermittent fasting (intermittent fasting). Picture this: instead of counting every calorie and agonizing over food choices around the clock, you focus on when you eat, not just what you eat. The simplicity of intermittent fasting lies in its adaptability to your daily life; it's a way of eating that cycles between controlled periods of eating and fasting. Unlike diet plans that can feel like wandering through a maze, intermittent fasting is like having a clear track to run on—less rules, more freedom.

Now, for a dose of science without the jargon—our bodies respond to eating and fasting by tapping into different fuel sources. When you eat, insulin levels rise, and your body goes into storage mode, saving some of that energy for later. But when you're fasting, insulin levels drop, and it's time for energy release. That's your body switching gears and burning fat for fuel. This is the crux of the fasting philosophy: allowing your body to efficiently alternate between these two states for optimal energy use and, yes, weight loss. But let's not jump ahead to the full story on metabolic enhancements and longevity—that's a treat reserved for the chapters to come. Instead, think of this chapter as your brisk morning stroll—an introduction to the fasting landscape that's ahead of us.

What about the notion that skipping meals leads to muscle loss, mood swings, and metabolism mayhem? That's another myth ready for busting. With intermittent fasting, we're not 'skipping' so much as strategically redirecting our eating schedules. This isn't about starvation; it's about harnessing the body's inherent mechanisms for managing energy. And for those wondering if fasting is another fad on the health horizon, rest assured, it's more than a mere trend. It's rooted in human history, woven into our very biology, and backed by modern science. We'll delve deeper into demystifying fasting myths soon enough. But for now, consider this a primer—a first peek into why traditional diets are losing grounds to the sustainable promise of a well-orchestrated fasting rhythm.

The Science of Intermittent Fasting

The enthralling concept of intermittent fasting isn't just a fleeting health trend; it's underpinned by a robust scientific foundation that is changing the way we think about eating and dieting. This section dives into the science behind why intermittent fasting isn't just another diet fad, but a shift in the paradigm that challenges traditional eating patterns and offers a refreshingly different perspective on how we can nurture our bodies.

At its core, intermittent fasting involves cycling between periods of eating and fasting. This isn't about depriving yourself; it's about reprogramming the timing and the 'when' of eating to allow your body to do what it does best—thrive. By strategically timing meals, we allow our body's inherent systems the time and space to perform intricate processes without the added burden of continuous digestion.

One of the key processes influenced by intermittent fasting is insulin sensitivity. Each time we consume food, particularly carbohydrates, our body's insulin levels rise to help shuttle glucose into cells for energy. By fasting, we reduce the constant spike of insulin, thereby helping to improve our body's sensitivity to it. Improved insulin sensitivity means less insulin is needed over time, which can lead to improved blood sugar control and reduced risk of developing type 2 diabetes.

While we're on the topic of hormones, let's not overlook the effects of intermittent fasting on growth hormone levels. Studies have shown that fasting can increase levels of this vitality-boosting hormone, which plays a pivotal role in muscle growth, metabolism, and fat burning. It's like hitting the body's reset button, giving it a chance to repair, rejuvenate, and burn fat more efficiently.

The science doesn't stop there. Autophagy is another biological process that's central to the science behind intermittent fasting. This is essentially the body's way of cleaning out damaged cells and regenerating new ones. When you fast, autophagy kicks into high gear, which could have profound implications for disease prevention and longevity—a topic we'll delve deeper into in later chapters.

But how can simply timing your eating patterns make such a difference? It all comes down to how our body uses energy. In the fed state, our body is digesting and absorbing food, primarily relying on glucose for energy. But when we fast, we burn through these glucose stores, and the body begins to break down fat for energy instead. This metabolic shift is often referred to as entering a state of ketosis, and it's a fundamental principle as to why intermittent fasting can be such an effective tool for weight loss.

Now, let's talk about the brain. Beyond the physical benefits, fasting has been shown to have promising effects on the brain's health and cognitive function. The brain-derived neurotrophic factor (BDNF) protein, which supports the survival of existing neurons and encourages the growth of new ones, is increased due to the stress that fasting places on the brain. In essence, what doesn't kill our cells, may indeed make them stronger.

Some may speculate that intermittent fasting could seem stressful to the body—and they're not entirely wrong. However, a fascinating aspect of intermittent fasting is the concept of hormesis: the idea that moderate stress can actually be beneficial. By challenging our cells just enough, we spur adaptations that ultimately lead to increased resilience and strength.

It's also worth noting the influence of intermittent fasting on our gut health. The gut microbiome is a bustling metropolis of bacteria that's crucial for our overall health. During fasting periods, the digestive system gets a much-needed rest, potentially lowering inflammation and allowing beneficial gut bacteria to thrive, thereby promoting healthy digestion and even improving mood and immune function.

In the context of weight loss, one cannot overlook the simplicity that intermittent fasting brings to calorie control. By condensing eating into shorter time frames, many people naturally eat less without the meticulous calorie counting that traditional diets often demand. It's a form of effort-less portion control, provided that when you do eat, you choose foods that are nutritious and satiating.

The ripple effects of intermittent fasting go beyond what we've covered thus far. For instance, the impact on cellular repair and metabolic health is profound. During fasting, cells activate pathways that not only help to break down and eliminate old and dysfunctional proteins, but also optimize energy metabolism, both of which are critical for maintaining health and preventing disease.

Still, fasting isn't just about the physical. It's about granting the body the opportunity to fall into its natural rhythm. Ancient humans didn't have access to supermarkets and food around the clock, and our bodies are likely optimized for periods of feasting and fasting—not constant food consumption. Many find that intermittent fasting helps to realign our bodies with a more ancestral eating pattern, which some suggest feels more natural and sustainable in the long run.

Understanding the science behind intermittent fasting is not just about appreciating its effects on weight loss, but its potential to revolutionize our relationship with food and health. When our bodies enter fasting states, they do remarkable things that can lead to a healthier, more vibrant life.

As we continue to explore the nuances of intermittent fasting, remember the science is clear: this isn't a mere diet, but a lifestyle that taps into our biology, empowering us to take back control over our health and wellbeing. With a little planning, patience, and knowledge, intermittent fasting might just be the keystone habit that can lead to lasting change.

As we wrap up this section on the science of intermittent fasting, it's important to appreciate the complexity and interconnectedness of the processes at work. Continued research will undoubtedly unveil even more about how this age-old practice affects our modern-day lives. In the coming chapters, we'll dissect some myths surrounding fasting, clarify its health benefits, tailor fasting plans to individual needs, and much more. Stay tuned as we delve deeper into making intermittent fasting a successful part of your lifestyle.

Demystifying Fasting Myths

The world of health and nutrition is often shrouded in a thick fog of myths and misunderstandings, particularly when it comes to the practice of intermittent fasting. Let's cut through that fog and shine a light on the facts. Dispelling these myths is crucial not only for knowledge's sake but also for helping individuals make informed decisions that could vastly improve their wellbeing.

One common myth suggests that fasting slows down metabolism, putting the body into starvation mode. This invokes images of a sluggish internal engine resisting weight loss efforts. However, research shows that short-term fasting actually increases metabolic rate, thanks to a surge in norepinephrine. The body, it seems, is not so easily fooled into thinking famine has struck.

Another prevalent fear is that muscle mass will waste away the moment we stop regular feeding. It's true that the body does need protein, but it doesn't mean it will immediately cannibalize muscle during a fast. The body is more adept at survival, using fat stores as the primary energy source during short-term fasts. It's a built-in efficiency system that evolution has honed over millennia.

Anxieties also circulate around the idea that skipping meals inevitably leads to overeating, turning fasting into a counterproductive endeavor. While binge eating is a risk if fasting is approached carelessly, conscious fasting teaches us to tune into real hunger cues. It can lead to better portion control in the long run.

Ever heard the one about breakfast being the most important meal of the day? It might be time to re-evaluate that axiom. While a morning meal can be beneficial for some, the rigid rule ignores our individual differences in metabolism and lifestyle. Focusing on nutrient density and eating in a window that suits your body's needs offers a more tailored way to thrive.

The concern that fasting must be painful and ridden with insatiable hunger is another myth to debunk. Initial hunger pangs may be more about habit than true hunger. Over time, the body adapts, and many practitioners report diminished hunger and even increased feelings of euphoria, thanks to ketone production.

Fearmongering voices often warn that fasting leads to nutrient deficiencies. However, if eating during non-fasting periods includes a variety of whole foods, your body will likely be well-nourished. Focusing on nutrient-dense foods during eating windows is essential.

Some argue fasting is just a fad. While the modern version comes with a hashtag and a community, the concept of intermittent fasting isn't new. It's been a practice in human cultures and various religions for centuries, used for health, spiritual, and practical reasons.

Concerns regarding fasting and low blood sugar often emerge, implying that without steady food intake, you'll inevitably crash. Again, the body is not that fragile. For the average non-diabetic individual, the liver is quite proficient at maintaining blood sugar levels within the normal range during fasting periods.

It's also widely believed that fasting is incompatible with a productive, energy-demanding life. However, many people find their cognition and energy levels actually increase after an adaptation period due to the enhanced release of adrenaline and improved neurological functioning.

Speaking of brain function, there's the persistent belief that fasting muddles your brain, clouding thought processes. The opposite is often true; fasting has been associated with clearer thinking and concentration, possibly due to ketones, which are known to be a more efficient fuel for the brain.

One of the most frustrating myths is that results from fasting are temporary. Sure, if someone reverts to unhealthy eating habits post-fasting, weight can return. But when viewed as a sustainable lifestyle change rather than a quick fix, intermittent fasting can help maintain healthy body weight along with numerous other health benefits.

Lastly, let's tackle the myth that fasting is dangerous. While there are certain scenarios where fasting isn't recommended, such as in pregnancy or certain health conditions, for the majority of people, intermittent fasting done correctly can be a safe and effective practice.

With myths like these cleared from the path, we can see intermittent fasting for what it truly is—a flexible, adaptable approach to eating that can suit a range of lifestyles and health goals. Don't let worn-out myths muddy the waters. The evidence is clear, and the potential benefits of intermittent fasting are too compelling to ignore.

Remember, like any lifestyle change, intermittent fasting should be approached with individualized consideration and, ideally, with guidance from healthcare professionals. Moving forward, let's arm ourselves with accurate information, attuned bodies, and open minds. Embracing fasting isn't about following a trend; it's about listening to science and potentially unlocking a more vibrant, health-aligned life.

Chapter 3

The Health Benefits Beyond the Scale

Shedding those pesky pounds is often the main attraction drawing many to the fasting spotlight, but what if I told you the real show begins when the weight loss curtain falls? The encores of intermittent fasting include a lineup of metabolic and cellular benefactors that might just steal the limelight. Metabolic enhancements, such as improved insulin sensitivity and reduced inflammation, aren't just backup singers to weight loss; they are headliners in their own right. Think about that for a second; your body could be humming a tune of health, with every cell dancing to a rhythm of rejuvenation.

Furthermore, fasting can crescendo into a symphony of longevity and disease prevention. It's like conducting your own internal orchestra, where each fasting period cues a series of biological processes that could help fend off chronic diseases. And then there's the piece de resistance: the potential to add years to your life. Now, that's something that deserves an encore! But let's not dive too deep into the hows and whys just yet—that's a performance reserved for the following subsections. Just know, that the fasting stage reveals more than a number twirling down on the scale; it's the whole health concert at play.

Stepping off the scale, you begin to see the full picture in all its glory. The spotlight shifts, and you realize you're not just aiming for a slimmer waistline but also for the boon of vigor and vitality that could very well rewrite the storyline of your golden years. It's not merely about taking a fleeting bow in a smaller pant size; it's about encores of wellness, standing ovations for your cells, and ultimately, a healthier, more vibrant you. And trust me, these are the kind of rave reviews you'll want to live for.

Metabolic Enhancements

Embarking on your journey into the world of intermittent fasting isn't solely a passport to weight loss. Still, it offers a cascade of benefits that ripple through every aspect of your metabolism. Have you ever pondered why some individuals seem to devour mountains of calories and never gain an ounce while others struggle to shed a single pound? The answer often lies within the efficiency of our metabolism. And guess what? Intermittent fasting can significantly enhance this metabolic efficiency.

Let's talk about what metabolism actually means. It's the complex web of processes by which your body converts food into energy. This isn't just about burning calories; it's about how your body manages all aspects of energy use and storage. Here's the kicker: intermittent fasting has been shown to tweak these metabolic processes in a way that could turn your body into a more efficient energy-managing powerhouse.

Do you often feel sluggish after meals, like you're running on low-grade fuel? This might be due to spikes in blood sugar levels, which can bog you down. Enter intermittent fasting, and you could well experience steadier energy levels. That's because your body begins to shift from relying on quick burns from sugars to tapping into your energy reserves—your fat stores. This gradual transition helps dodge those post-meal crashes and keeps you laser-focused and full of vim throughout your day.

It's not just about feeling good. In a well-nourished fasted state, your body does a marvelous thing: it starts to clean house. Autophagy, a process we'll get into in more detail another time, is your body's way of clearing out damaged cells to make way for new ones. It's like hitting the reset button on your cellular health, and it takes the fast to flip the switch.

And then there's insulin, a hormone that plays a prime role in your metabolic performance. When you fast intermittently, you give your body a chance to lower its insulin levels, which helps prevent insulin resistance. Why is that important? Because insulin resistance is often the gateway to a slew of metabolic disorders. Simply put, having your body more attuned to insulin means the food you eat is less likely to be stored as fat and more likely to be used as fuel.

Another metabolic perk to add to your list is increased human growth hormone (HGH) levels. This is the stuff of youth, the hormone that plays a key role in growth, metabolism, and muscle strength. Who knew that the fountain of youth might not be a potion or a pill, but a strategically timed schedule of eating and fasting? Intermittent fasting can boost your HGH, keeping you feeling and functioning youthfully.

Your liver is your unsung metabolic hero, and it loves intermittent fasting. When you fast, your liver converts body fat into ketones—a clean, high-octane fuel for your body. The process of entering ketosis enhances brain health and energy levels while also contributing to reduced inflammation throughout the body. It's like upgrading your body's fuel from regular unleaded to premium!

Cholesterol and heart health are also beneficiaries of intermittent fasting's metabolic enhancements. Surprising, isn't it? By moderating the window in which you eat, you can improve your lipid profile. This means potentially lower LDL ("bad" cholesterol) levels and higher HDL ("good" cholesterol) levels. It's like turning the tides on cholesterol buildup, keeping your arteries more like open highways than congested byways.

Fatty liver disease, a rising concern in the health community, may also be assuaged through intermittent fasting. By curtailing the influx of dietary fats and sugars that your liver must process, you give it time to break down fat stores and decrease the accumulation of fat in your liver cells. It's almost as if each fast gives your liver a mini detox.

Amplifying the effects of intermittent fasting is exercise. Regular physical activity dovetails beautifully with your fasting regimen, increasing the rate and efficiency of metabolic enhancements. This synergy cultivates an environment where fat loss isn't just probable—it's expected.

What about the perils of diets that depress your metabolism, causing weight loss to stagnate? Intermittent fasting sidesteps this often demoralizing effect. Instead of continually cutting calories, which can cause your body's metabolism to downshift, intermittent fasting intermittently revs up your metabolic engine. The result? You keep burning at a high gear without the plateau.

Feeling hot? That might be your body's thermogenesis at work—a fancy term for heat production. Intermittent fasting can elevate thermogenesis, contributing to your body's ability to burn calories as heat rather than store them. Imagine a fireplace inside you, steadily burning off what you consume for that satisfying cozy warmth—that's thermogenesis.

And let's not overlook the realm of gut health. Your digestive system is a labyrinth of happenings that impact your overall metabolism. Intermittent fasting can enhance gut health by promoting diverse gut flora and giving your digestive system much-needed downtime to repair and recover. This isn't just good news for your stomach, but for your entire body's metabolic network.

Lastly, the beauty of intermittent fasting in the context of metabolic enhancement is that it's adaptable. Whether you're an early riser or a night owl, you can mold your fasting schedule to suit your body's natural rhythm. By aligning fasting with your circadian cycle, your metabolism doesn't just steadily burn—it dances to your individual biological beat.

Understanding the metabolic enhancements afforded by intermittent fasting equips you with the hardy tools needed to not just lose weight but transform your entire body's functioning. It's less about the number on the scale and more about under-the-hood improvements that ultimately lead to a healthier, energized, and revitalized you. As you turn the page, remember that embracing intermittent fasting is much like engaging in any great endeavor—it's a commitment to igniting the very best version of your metabolic self.

Longevity and Disease Prevention

When we shift our focus beyond the digits on the scale, we open up a world where the benefits of intermittent fasting extend into the golden years of life, casting a protective net against a myriad of health conditions. This section delves into how intermittent fasting isn't just about fitting into a smaller clothes size—it's about wrapping your future self in a layer of health and vitality.

We've seen how intermittent fasting can aid in metabolism enhancement, but its role in longevity and disease prevention is where it truly shines. Our bodies are crafted to last, to endure, and fasting is akin to a tune-up for a machine, ensuring that the gears continue to turn smoothly and efficiently as years pass by.

Those within the bandwidth of 21 to 75 years old are often caught in the whirlwind of life where the health choices made today lay the bricks for the road ahead. How does intermittent fasting pave this road to being more robust and disease resistant? It starts at the cellular level.

Consider the process of autophagy, where the cells clean house, recycling old and damaged components. intermittent fasting triggers this cellular 'spring cleaning,' so to speak. This mechanism is like giving your cells the opportunity to renew themselves, potentially delaying the aging process and reducing the risk of disease by keeping cellular debris at a minimum.

Furthermore, fasting has a profound impact on your body's inflammation levels. Chronic inflammation is like a silent alarm going off constantly, eventually contributing to various diseases such as diabetes, heart conditions, and even cancer. intermittent fasting, by reducing inflammation, could be akin to quieting this alarm, creating an environment where diseases struggle to take root.

Linked to inflammation is the role of oxidative stress in the body, a scenario where free radicals, those unstable atoms, run amok, potentially leading to chronic diseases and aging. The fasting state encourages the body to bolster its defenses, increasing antioxidant activities and enhancing your body's ability to combat this oxidative stress.

The big 'C', cardiovascular disease, stands as one of the most common foes in the narrative of human health. Intermittent fasting steps onto the scene here, showing promise in improving blood pressure, cholesterol levels, and triglycerides—all key actors in the drama of heart health. By casting intermittent fasting in a lead role, we could be looking at a way to potentially reduce the prevalence of heart disease.

When we talk about sugars and fats, we often only consider their impact on waistlines. Yet, these molecules play a pivotal role in the development of metabolic conditions like type 2 diabetes. intermittent fasting emerges as a protagonist by improving insulin sensitivity and altering the body's relationship with glucose. This new script means lower blood sugar levels and a reduced risk of becoming diabetic.

But let's not forget the most magnificent organ in the body—the brain. Cognitive function and neurological health are paramount, and intermittent fasting demonstrates its versatility by promoting brain health. It's like a mental gym for your neurons, fostering the growth of new nerve cells, and it may enhance brain function, potentially protecting against neurodegenerative diseases like Alzheimer's and Parkinson's.

Cancer, the word itself evokes fear, but fasting brings a glimmer of hope. By altering the metabolic pathways that cancer cells thrive on, intermittent fasting might just lower the incidence of cancer. It starves cancer cells by depriving them of the constant supply of fuel they need to grow, offering a fresh perspective on cancer prevention strategies.

Even the bones that scaffold our very essence benefit from intermittent fasting. There's evidence suggesting that fasting can bolster bone density, orchestrating a stronger framework for the body to weather the storms of the later years, and reducing the chance of osteoporosis and fractures.

An added boon of intermittent fasting is its potential to attune the body's response to stress at a cellular level. Heat shock proteins increase, molecular chaperones protect cells, and cellular stress resistance skyrockets. It's akin to training your cells in self-defense against the assaults of aging and disease.

In the context of longevity and disease prevention, the merits of intermittent fasting become a symphony orchestrating a state of well-being that extends beyond the present moment. It's about creating a sanctuary for your health where time's natural erosion is slowed, its impact more graceful, its stamp less severe. By choosing the path of intermittent fasting, you aren't just changing your now; you're investing in the wealth of your years to come, ensuring that every heartbeat and every breath takes you further along a journey of sustained good health.

Let's embrace intermittent fasting not only to achieve and maintain a healthy weight but to gift ourselves with the potential for a longer, more robust life. It's about putting a stake in the ground for the future, a future filled with possibility, vitality, and health, making every day count toward building a lasting legacy of wellness.

In closing this chapter on longevity and disease prevention, remember that the choices you make on your eating and fasting schedule today echo into the corridors of your future. It's not just about surviving; it's about thriving. With intermittent fasting, you have a potent tool at your disposal to help you do just that.

Chapter 4

Finding Your Fasting Rhythm

As we turn the page from understanding the health perks that tag along with intermittent fasting, let's focus our attention on nailing down your personal fasting groove. The search for the ideal fasting window is not a one-size-fits-all affair. It's about tuning into your body's unique tempo and crafting a schedule that harmonizes effortlessly with your daily life. Think of it as a dance between your body's innate patterns and your lifestyle needs. Whether it's the hustle of early mornings or the quiet of late evenings that you resonate with, your fasting rhythm can mold around the contours of your routine, empowering not just weight loss, but a symphony of wellness benefits without missing a beat.

Let's clear the floor for some real talk—finding that sweet spot, your individualized fasting cadence, requires some introspection. It's about observing how your energy ebbs and flows throughout the day and aligning your fasting window to amplify those natural highs and cushion the lows. Say you're an early riser who hits the ground running at dawn; an early fasting window may work wonders for your metabolic vigor. Or perhaps you're a night owl, your creativity sparking after dark; a later eating window might play to your strengths. Trust your body's signals—they're the most authentic cues to identifying a fasting schedule that feels as natural as breathing.

And it's not just about the clock ticking away. Adjusting the intensity of your fasting is akin to setting the volume on a speaker—just right for your ears. Are you the type who dives in headfirst, or do you prefer dipping your toes into the water to test the temperature? Your fasting protocol can and should adjust to your personal comfort level, be it a gentle 12-hour overnight reset or a more challenging 24-hour cleanse. The goal isn't to plunge into the deep end immediately but to wade in gradually, ensuring the experience resonates with your body's needs and your mind's resolve. Staying flexible, patient and listening to the subtle whisperings of your body, you'll be well on your way to striking that perfect fasting harmony.

Understanding Circadian Rhythms

Embarking on a journey to understand intermittent fasting isn't just about skipping meals—it's comprehending the symphony of biological processes that work in harmony with the earth's 24-hour cycle. This cyclical daily pattern, known as the circadian rhythm, isn't just about when we feel sleepy or awake. It's intricately linked to how our body functions, including digestion, metabolism, and even how we process nutrients.

Grasping the circadian rhythm concept is like discovering the conductor of an orchestra. Without the conductor's guidance, the musical ensemble would falter—a similar scenario unfolds in our bodies when our internal rhythms are out of sync. Think of each cell in your body like a musician with its own instrument, playing to the beat directed by the circadian rhythm.

Our internal clock is primarily regulated by light. When sunlight enters our eyes, it signals our brain to stay awake and alert. As dusk falls, the absence of light cues the production of melatonin, coaxing our body into sleep mode. But it doesn't stop at sleep; this rhythm influences our hormones, eating habits, and ultimately, the way we metabolize food.

If we're munching on a midnight snack while our body is winding down, we're essentially asking the digestive system to hit a high note in the middle of a soft melody. This off-tune snacking can cause our metabolism to stutter, making weight loss more elusive than ever. It's no wonder that the traditional eat-whenever-you-want diet often misses a key performance—timing.

Consider the power of aligning fasting with our circadian rhythms. It means we eat when our body is at its metabolic peak, taking full advantage of our natural digestive abilities. Conversely, we fast during our body's downtime, allowing for rest and repair. This isn't just a theory; numerous studies demonstrate how eating in tune with our circadian rhythm can lead to better weight management and overall health.

Yet, there's a rub. Our modern lifestyle often competes with our natural circadian preferences. We're exposed to artificial light late into the night, work shifts that jumble our sleep patterns, and have 24/7 access to food. Resetting our body's clock to its natural rhythm may seem daunting in such a context. However, it's a challenge well worth taking on.

Embracing fasting within the context of circadian rhythms means understanding that timing is not just a detail—it's a critical component of the strategy. Remember, it's not only what you eat but when you eat that matters. By synchronizing meal patterns with our body clock, we support our natural cycles of fasting and eating, which can lead to more effective weight loss and improved metabolic health.

Naturally, there's individual variation in how each person's circadian rhythm functions, and this dictates the best times to eat and fast. Some of us are larks, rising with the sun and functioning best in the morning, while others are night owls, coming alive as the day wanes. Recognizing which type you are can help tune your fasting schedule for optimum results.

A circadian-aligned fasting schedule often involves finishing your last meal in the early evening and fasting overnight until breakfast the next morning. This period of fasting aligns with your body's natural inclination to repair and rejuvenate during sleep. By extending this fasting state, you extend the period of restorative work your body performs.

Let's not forget the hormonal dance that accompanies our circadian rhythms. Insulin sensitivity, for instance, tends to be higher earlier in the day and declines as night approaches. This means your body is better equipped to handle carbohydrates and sugars in the earlier part of the day compared to the evening. Properly timing your fast can capitalize on this daily hormonal ebb and flow.

So, how do you start realigning your eating patterns with your circadian rhythms? Begin by observing the natural cues your body offers—when do you feel hungry, when does your energy peak, and when do you feel ready to wind down? These signals help craft a fasting plan that feels almost second nature because it's designed to work with, not against, your body's inherent rhythms.

An aligned circadian fasting approach is not just about losing weight. It's about fostering an environment where your body can thrive—mitigating inflammation, bolstering cell repair, and even improving mental clarity. It's recognizing that our bodies have evolved to operate in a certain rhythm, finely tuned to the cycles of day and night.

Finally, while it's crucial to honor our circadian rhythms, there's also room for flexibility. Life happens, and there will be days when late dinners or early breakfasts are unavoidable. The key is to aim for consistency without becoming rigid. Your fasting journey should enhance your life, not become another source of stress.

Understanding circadian rhythms isn't merely an academic exercise—it's a transformational tool. It empowers you to synchronize your fasting practice with the natural tempo of your body, turning the tide in your favor in the quest for sustainable weight loss and profound well-being. It's the secret ingredient that might just unlock the potential you've been waiting to unleash.

Personalizing Your Fasting Plan

With the foundation of intermittent fasting principles securely in place, it's time to sculpt a fasting plan that feels as though it's tailored just for you. Think of your body as a unique ecosystem, operating under its own rules, rhythms, and responses. From your sleeping patterns to your work schedule, every aspect can influence how you fast. While some thrive on an early window, greeting the sunrise with nourishment and closing the kitchen by afternoon, others find solace in an evening meal shared with loved ones. It's not just about when you eat; it's also about understanding the dance between intensity and sustainability. Your body's whisperings are there to guide you; an energy dip here, a sleep disturbance there, these signs help you determine the right fasting intensity for you. Whether it's easing into a 16-hour fast or comfortably pushing to a 24-hour reset, your fasting plan isn't static—it evolves, bends and blossoms with you. So let's cast aside the one-size-fits-all diet mentality and embark on a journey of self-discovery, where you become the architect of your fasting plan, carefully listening to and nurturing your body's own wisdom for lasting transformation.

Tailoring the Timing: Successful intermittent fasting isn't one-size-fits-all; it involves syncing your eating patterns with your individual lifestyle and biological cues. When it comes to the timing of your fasting and eating windows, a tailored approach can make all the difference between a regimen that feels like an uphill battle and one that smoothly integrates with your life.

Consider the fact that everyone's daily schedules vary greatly. A night shift worker, for instance, will have a vastly different timetable than someone working a 9-5 job. The beauty of intermittent fasting is that it's adaptable. It can be shifted and shaped to fit around your particular routine, so you don't have to revamp your entire life to accommodate your eating patterns.

Take circadian rhythms into account. Your body's natural sleep-wake cycles influence your metabolism, and aligning your fasting schedule with these rhythms can enhance the benefits of your fasting plan. For many, this might mean refraining from eating late at night and breaking their fast in the morning or early afternoon, thus tapping into the body's innate propensity for daytime activity and nighttime rest.

When considering how to tailor the timing of your fasting, listen to your hunger cues. Initiating your fasting period when you're typically less hungry can make the process feel much more manageable. If you're not a breakfast person, skip it without guilt and begin eating later in the day. If dinner isn't as important to you, consider an earlier eating window.

Your energy levels throughout the day can also guide the timing of your meals. Some people find that they are most alert and productive with a hearty lunch and a light dinner. Others may discover that a solid breakfast provides the necessary fuel for their day. Use these natural ebbs and flows of energy to decide when to eat and when to fast.

Digestive comfort is crucial as well—ending your eating window at least a couple of hours before bedtime can lead to better sleep and a more restful fasting period. Lying down shortly after eating can be uncomfortable and disruptive to sleep, so plan your last meal to give yourself some digestive downtime.

Also, take into account your workout schedule. Exercising while in a fasted state can bolster fat loss and energy utilization, but this needs to be carefully timed so you're not left feeling depleted. Conversely, if you like to eat pre-workout for energy, make sure that it aligns with your eating window.

For those with a family or social life that revolves around evening meals, your fasting schedule might look different. Perhaps a later eating window allows you to engage in those dinner gatherings without feeling excluded or compromising your goals. Here is where the flexibility of intermittent fasting shines, and it's vital to mold your plan to fit your social life, not the other way around.

If you have medical conditions that require timing certain medications with food, this too will influence your fasting schedule. Always consult with a healthcare provider to ensure that any fasting regimen you adopt is safe and effective, given your specific health circumstances.

Remember, the length of your fast is flexible. While some may thrive on a 16-hour fast, others might find their sweet spot at 12 hours or extend it to 20. Initially, experimentation is key to determining what feels best for your body. Track your responses to different fasting windows to identify the most suitable pattern for your lifestyle.

Adjusting to a new fasting schedule may require patience. Your body might need time to adapt to different meal timing, and that's perfectly normal. Initial feelings of hunger or discomfort should subside as your body becomes accustomed to your personalized fasting rhythm.

The frequency of your fasts also plays a role in your scheduling. Some may choose to fast daily, while others might opt for alternate-day fasting or less frequent 24-hour fasts. Consider how often you want to incorporate fasting and what timing aligns with that choice.

Lastly, be mindful of periods of higher stress or lack of sleep, which might affect your ability to maintain a strict fasting schedule. During these times, it could be wise to shorten your fasting period or adjust your eating window to provide more flexibility and support to your body.

Ultimately, tailoring the timing to suit your unique circumstances isn't just about making intermittent fasting work for you; it's about creating a sustainable lifestyle change that encourages balance and wellness. When the fasting schedule you choose feels natural, you are well on your way to discovering the secret behind lasting weight loss success.

As you explore this process, remember that flexibility and adaptability are your allies. Be willing to modify your approach as your life's demands evolve, ensuring that your intermittent fasting practice is always working for your highest benefit—a harmony between health goals and life's pleasures.

Adjusting the Intensity: As you find your fasting rhythm, you'll discover the need to tweak the intensity of your fasting plan. This isn't a matter of mere preference; it's a strategic move to maximize benefits while ensuring your body and mind can sustain this transformative lifestyle. Internally, your body will communicate, through various signals, when it's time to ramp up the intensity or scale it back. It's on you to listen wisely.

So, what does "adjusting the intensity" entail in the context of intermittent fasting? Essentially, it's the ebb and flow of how challenging your fasting periods are. This might mean lengthening the duration of your fasts or altering the frequency, depending on what your body requires and can handle at any given phase in your journey.

For beginners, starting with a gentle approach is usually encouraged. Ease into intermittent fasting with shorter fasting windows like the 12:12 or the 16:8 method—the hours represent your fasting and feeding periods, respectively. This acclimatization phase isn't just about physical adaptation; it's about mental preparation too. Both your body and mind need this time to understand and embrace the shifts that are taking place.

Now, as you progress, you'll possibly find that these windows are no longer challenging. That's a signal to up the ante. But how do you know it's the right time? Listen to your body. Are you sailing through 16-hour fasts without a second thought? Are hunger pangs now practically non-existent? You might be ready to extend your fasting window to 18 or even 20 hours.

And then there's the aspect of intensity that's beyond the clock. Some endure their fasts with nothing but water, while others allow for black coffee or tea. If you're incorporating these non-caloric drinks into your fasting window and find the experience too comfortable, or if your weight loss has plateaued, consider purifying your fast to water only.

Feeling a bit apprehensive about intensifying your fast? That's a normal reaction. Take this as your cue to approach changes incrementally. There's no need to jump from a 16:8 to a one-day water fast straight away. Nudge your fasting window an hour at a time, or experiment with a 24-hour fast once a week to start.

Don't forget that fasting is not just about the absence of food but also about the presence of mindfulness when it comes to eating. Adjusting the intensity could mean becoming more stringent with your eating windows. Ensure you're not overcompensating during those times, which can be easy to do after a long fast. Pay attention to your body's satiety signals even when not fasting.

Intensity, of course, doesn't imply recklessness. If you ever feel unwell or too strained, it's essential to scale back. Intermittent fasting isn't about pushing through pain or ignoring the warning signs your body sends you. It's about challenging yourself within the bounds of what is beneficial and sustainable for you.

Balancing fasting intensity also matters when life throws curveballs. Stressful periods, whether emotional, physical, or psychological, may warrant a reduction in fasting intensity. During such times, your body will need more energy to cope, and it's perfectly fine to shorten your fasting windows or relax your rules around them.

Remember, the goal of adjusting the intensity isn't to compete with others or even with your past self. It's to find what works for you now, laying a sustainable path for continual improvement and adaptation.

On the technical side, how do you measure the results of intensity adjustments? Keeping a fasting journal can be immensely helpful. Note how you felt during and after changes to your fasting schedule. Has your energy improved? Any changes in mood or sleep patterns? These observations will steer you toward the perfect balance.

Moreover, consistently tracking your progress extends beyond self-observation. Using apps or tools that monitor your fasting hours and feeding habits gives you a visual representation of the journey. It's not just about weight; pay attention to other health markers like blood pressure or blood sugar levels, as they can be indicative of your fasting intensity's effectiveness.

In the end, adjusting the intensity of your intermittent fasting plan is a highly personal process. What's essential is that you remain flexible and responsive to your body's needs, using intermittent fasting as a tool to reach not only your weight loss goals but to enhance your overall health and well-being.

As you become more adept at fasting, you might be tempted to test the waters with more advanced methods, like alternate-day fasting or the 5:2 diet. But, let's save that for when you're truly ready and have mastered the art of adjusting the intensity. Until then, focus on finding that sweet spot where challenge and comfort intersect, paving the way for a sustainable and health-aligned fasting experience.

In concluding this section, remember: adjusting the intensity is an ongoing conversation with your body, an open dialogue about what you need to thrive. Stay attuned to the messages your body sends, and don't be afraid to make the necessary adjustments. Your perseverance, coupled with intelligent adaptation, is what will ultimately drive your success in intermittent fasting and beyond.

Chapter 5

The Psychology of Fasting

Embarking on a journey with intermittent fasting isn't just about changing what or when you eat; it's a profound psychological leap into reprogramming how you think about food and hunger. The mind, a beautiful, complex, and often obstinate entity, can be your greatest ally or your fiercest opponent. Imagine reframing your hunger, not as a dreaded enemy, but as a gentle reminder of your body's natural fasting rhythm. It's about understanding that hunger isn't perpetual but comes in waves, and each wave you surf brings you closer to your goal. Fasting instills a sense of empowerment, allowing you to take back control and listen to your body's true needs rather than the arbitrary eating schedule society has prescribed.

As you stand at this crossroads, remember that overcoming psychological barriers can be thought of as the mental 'muscle-building' part of your fasting regimen. It's common to encounter mental resistance, rooted in years of conditioned habits and emotional eating patterns. Yet, with each fasting interval, these mental barriers become less daunting. You develop resilience not just in your body, but in your mind too. Just as muscles strengthen with exercise, your ability to maintain your fasting protocol will grow more robust, transforming what once felt like an internal tug-of-war into a harmonious dance with your physiological cues.

Why does this matter? Because the success of your fasting journey hinges not only on your body's biological response, but equally on your mental fortitude. The intrinsic motivation, the psychological 'why' behind your choice to fast, has to be crystal clear to weather the periods of adjustment. When you anticipate and navigate the psychological currents of fasting with intention and awareness, you're not just losing weight; you're gaining insights into your own behavioral patterns and potential. That's a transformative experience, one that transcends the confines of diet culture and propels you into a realm of lasting, sustainable change.

The Mental Shift

Embarking on a journey of intermittent fasting isn't simply about scheduling meals; it's fundamentally a mental marathon. Those who succeed in fasting don't just alter their eating windows—they instigate a profound mental shift, reinterpreting hunger, self-control, and the role food plays in their lives. Approaching fasting with the right mindset is half the battle, and possibly the most critical part of the process.

Picture this: a life where you're no longer chained to the clock for your next meal, where you're liberated from the constant cycle of snacking and digesting. This isn't a fantasy; it's the mental reorientation that fasting can bring. Instead of food controlling you, you gain control over food. The mental shift allows you to understand that feelings of hunger aren't emergencies; they're simply signals, and ones that our bodies are well-equipped to handle.

Let's talk about the empowerment that fasting brings—once embraced, it shatters the previously held notion that you need to eat three square meals a day, or that snacks are necessary to tide you over. Knowledge is power, and understanding the physiological underpinnings of fasting can embolden you to face hunger head-on, recognizing it as a sign that your body is switching gears to burn fat as fuel.

Food, for so many, is a source of comfort and pleasure. When adopting a fasting lifestyle, it's not just the routine of eating that changes, but your relationship with food as well. One begins to appreciate the quality over quantity, learning that what you eat matters profoundly more than how often you eat. It's a renaissance of culinary appreciation—you start to savor flavors, textures, and the joy of nourishing the body appropriately.

Resistance to habitual patterns is natural. We've been conditioned to crave instant gratification, but fasting teaches patience and appreciation for delayed satisfaction. It's not about starving or deprivation—it's about waiting for what you truly want. And often, you may find that after a fast, what you thought you craved isn't quite what your body needs.

This mental shift isn't without its challenges. Social pressures, ingrained beliefs, and the habitual comfort of routines can often create a gravitational pull back to the old ways. But those who navigate this transition recognize the brief discomfort as the birth pains of a new, healthier lifestyle. Consistency and a steadfast focus on the end goal fortify the mental resolve.

Imagine the freedom of not being a slave to cravings. When you decouple emotional needs from nutritional ones, you unlock a level of bodily autonomy many can hardly dream of. This doesn't happen overnight, but with time, the fasting mindset becomes second nature, and that doughnut or bag of chips loses its siren call.

One of the most enormous shifts occurs in the perception of hunger. Many fear hunger as if it were a monster lurking around the corner. But through the practice of fasting, you will likely discover that hunger comes in waves and recedes just as naturally if you don't immediately feed it. Learning to ride these waves can be an empowering experience, demonstrating your inner strength and diminishing the tyrannical hold hunger once had over you.

With fasting, you also start to see the body's signaling systems for what they are—a dialogue between your physiology and your environment. You become attuned to what genuine hunger signals are, as opposed to boredom or stress-induced eating cues. It's like learning a new language to converse harmoniously with your body.

Don't mistake this mental shift as merely a psychological strategy—it leads to behavioral changes that align with your health goals. By changing your outlook on fasting and hunger, you set yourself up for success because you believe in the process, not just as a dieting technique, but as a lifestyle upgrade that reverberates through every facet of your life.

This mindset transformation also encapsulates the understanding of the impermanence of eating pleasures compared to the lasting benefits of health and vitality. The short-lived pleasure of eating frequently or indulging cannot compare with the profound and enduring sense of well-being that comes from a body that's been given the respite it deserves through fasting.

A mental shift also involves recognizing the misinformation that's often peddled by food companies and diet trends. With the clarity that fasting brings, you begin to see through the marketing hype and make food choices based on nutritional value and personal health goals rather than advertising. It's about becoming a savvy consumer and a custodian of your health.

It's also important to acknowledge that with this mental shift, it's not about being perfect. It's about progress, understanding, and forgiveness. Slips will happen, old habits die hard, but each time you fast, you reinforce the mental armor against the cultural tide of constant consumption. You'll find that as your fasting practice deepens, so does your mental resilience.

Finally, this shift is where the magic of fasting truly lies—it's in the mental fortitude that says, 'I am in control, not my hunger,' and 'My body is a temple, and I choose when to nourish it.' With this mentality, fasting evolves from a dieting tactic to a transformative life practice. Your body's needs, your mind's resolve, and an unwavering commitment to well-being become the symphony that guides your daily choices, and ultimately, leads you to a robust, healthier life.

And therein lies the secret sauce—when the mental shift takes hold, the true potential of intermittent fasting emerges. It's no longer a chore, a mere method, or a trend. It becomes a conscious choice for self-improvement, a statement of how you value your health, and a testament to the strength of your will. Prepare to take the reins of your health journey firmly in hand as you redefine your relationship with food and embrace the empowering practice of fasting.

DAVID ALEXANDER

Overcoming Psychological Barriers

As we unpack the myriad aspects entangling our relationship with food, we recognize that mastering the mental game is often half the battle when venturing into the world of fasting. It's not unusual to be trapped by psychological barriers that distort our perspective on hunger and satiation. Pushing past these mental barricades requires strategy, not just willpower. Let's navigate through these and explore how breaking free can unlock fasting's full potential.

Embrace the idea that hunger isn't an emergency. We've long been wired to respond to the slightest grumble in our stomachs as if it's a five-alarm fire. This sensation isn't a danger signal; it's simply a natural bodily cue. Realizing that you won't wither away from feeling hungry for a bit is critical. With time and practice, these feelings will not only become less intimidating but also more manageable.

Recognize fasting as a skill that can be honed rather than an innate trait you're born with – or without. Much like learning to play an instrument or mastering a new language, getting better at fasting comes with consistent, mindful practice. Patience is key. As you become more accustomed to the ebb and flow of your fasting routine, what once seemed daunting will slowly become second nature.

Identify and confront the emotional ties we have with eating. Our lives are often punctuated with food-centric celebrations, comfort eating, and sometimes mindless snacking during periods of boredom or stress. Acknowledging these patterns without judgment is the first step toward untangling the hold they may have over our eating habits. Understanding

50

what triggers these responses can help us reroute our impulses during a fast.

Set clear, achievable goals, and celebrate the milestones along the way. Small victories are the stepping stones to long-term success. Redirect the focus from what you're 'missing out on' to the progress you're making. Each hour you successfully fast, every temptation you bypass is a triumph and should be regarded as such.

Learn to differentiate between physical hunger and psychological craving. This can be a game-changer. When the thought of food encroaches upon your focus, question whether your body truly needs nourishment or if it's simply a habitual desire. Once you can make this distinction, you'll find that many hunger pangs during a fast are not emergencies, but mere whispers that can be hushed with mindfulness and hydration.

Visualize success. This technique isn't just for athletes. Imagining yourself completing a fast and reaping the benefits primes your subconscious for success. It also strengthens your resolve when you encounter inevitable rough patches along the journey. Visualization helps in building a resilient mindset that's attuned to achievement rather than apprehension.

Commune with others on the same path. A support system can bolster your determination. Share experiences and advice with fasting groups or friends who engage in similar lifestyle changes. Knowing that you're not alone in your endeavor makes the process less daunting, and can breathe new life into your resolve when it's flickering.

Mitigate stress with meditation or other calming practices. Stress can be a relentless saboteur of fasting goals. It amplifies cravings and masks the mental clarity fasting brings. Tapping into practices that foster peace can help clear mental clutter that triggers stress-eating and weakens fasting discipline.

Foster a sense of curiosity about your body's signals. Instead of dreading hunger, approach it as a researcher would: observe, take notes, and be curious. This shifts your perspective from one of avoidance to one of interest. How does hunger feel at different times? How does it come and go? This can lead to a richer understanding of your relationship with food and fasting.

Maintain flexibility in your approach. Rigidity can breed a sense of failure when plans go awry. Life is unpredictable, and so is fasting. Adopt an adaptable mindset where deviations aren't seen as failures, but rather parts of the journey. Flexibility can prevent despondency and keep you on the path without undue self-reproach.

Nourish your mind. During fasting periods, engage in activities that stimulate and consume your attention, rather than those that leave room for food-focused thoughts to creep in. Whether it's dabbling in a hobby, diving into work, or losing yourself in a book, keep your cognitive space filled with enriching experiences.

Addressing the inevitable plateau with a tactical pause rather than despair is essential. Plateaus are not dead ends; they're just the body's way of recalibrating. Use this time to reassess, make necessary adjustments and acknowledge the progress you've made thus far.

Celebrate non-scale victories. It's common to become fixated on the numbers on the scale, but the benefits of fasting extend beyond weight. Celebrate improved mental clarity, increased energy, and a better relationship with food. When you learn to appreciate these intangible rewards, you fuel your motivation even more.

Enlist the help of technology. Use apps and tools to track your fasting periods, your moods, and your wins. These can serve as reminders of how far you've come and can help keep you strategically aligned with your goals. Just as we use maps to navigate unfamiliar terrain, these resources guide us through the psychological landscape of fasting.

Lastly, resist the tendency to rush the process. Our brains need time to rewire old habits and forge new pathways. Much like physical exercise, the mental exercise of fasting strengthens with time and consistency. Keep at it, and trust that the psychological barriers you face today will become the milestones of your fasting wisdom tomorrow.

Chapter 6

Nutritional Strategies for Effective Fasting

As we've delved into the intricacies of intermittent fasting, it's clear that this isn't just about skipping meals, but about smart strategies that boost your results. In this chapter, you'll learn that what you eat is just as critical as when you eat. Consider this: your nutritional approach during your eating windows can either catapult your progress or drag you down. That's why we're zeroing in on eating for success – it's about making every calorie count. Nourishing your body with the right foods ensures you receive all the essential nutrients, keeping you robust and satiated during your fasts. It's not just about reducing the frequency of your meals but also enhancing their quality. High-density, nutrient-rich meals become your allies, delivering sustained energy and preventing those all-too-familiar diet downfalls.

So, how do you construct a feast that adds momentum to your fasting efforts? It's about striking a fine balance. Lean proteins, healthy fats, and complex carbohydrates can't be overlooked. They're your body's building blocks, creating a well-oiled machine that thrives during periods of fasting. And let's not forget fiber. This unsung hero doesn't just aid digestion; it's a heavyweight champion in the ring, battling hunger pangs and stabilizing blood sugar levels. Sprinkled judiciously throughout your diet, these components serve to amplify your body's fasting potential. Think of it as fine-tuning an engine – with the right fuel, you'll run smoothly and efficiently, burning through reserves, rather than sputtering out halfway through the race.

Nutritional strategies are central, not peripheral, to a successful fasting regimen. You'll find that tapping into powerful food synergy can provide an astonishing uplift to your fasting journey. But here's the kicker – these aren't just nutritionists' best-kept secrets or unfounded claims. These strategies are backed by a burgeoning body of research pointing to the profound impact that a well-curated diet has on fasting efficacy. The mindful selection of foods bursting with vitamins and minerals can help to maintain muscle mass, bolster immune function, and stave off cravings. Keep in mind that intermittent fasting isn't a one-size-fits-all venture. Your nutritional needs are unique, so a dash of personalization will serve you well in crafting a plan that's tailored to your lifestyle – ensuring your fasting story is one of triumph, not trial.

Eating for Success

Now that we've entered the realm of intermittent fasting, there's a pivotal component we need to tackle: eating for success. The meals you have during your eating windows are not just about satisfying hunger—they're about nurturing your body, optimizing your fast, and laying the groundwork for a sustainable lifestyle change.

Think of your eating window as prime time for nutrition. It's not just about what tastes good; it's about what fuels your body for both the fasting period and your overall health. This means selecting nutrient-dense foods that provide energy, support metabolism, and maintain muscle mass. It's about quality over quantity, every single time.

Balance is key. Don't think you need to feast like royalty every time you break a fast. Instead, break your fast gently. Start with something light like a salad or broth-based soup. These foods are easy on your digestive system and prepare your body for the upcoming nutrients without causing an overload.

Hydration is crucial, too. You might think fasting is just about the food, but what you drink plays an integral role. Water, herbal teas, and electrolyte-rich beverages can support your fast by keeping you hydrated and making the fasting period smoother.

One common misconception is that you can eat anything within your eating window. It's essential to understand that binging on junk foods can negate the benefits of your fast. Focus on whole foods—lean proteins, heart-healthy fats, fiber-rich carbohydrates, and plenty of fruits and vegetables.

Aiming for diversity in your meals not only keeps things interesting but also ensures a wide range of vitamins and minerals. You don't need to be a top chef to whip up nourishing meals; simplicity often leads to the greatest nutritional success. Grilled fish, a rainbow of vegetables, a drizzle of olive oil—these simple ingredients create a powerhouse plate.

Let's tap into the nuts and bolts of macronutrients. Proteins, for example, are essential during your eating periods. They're the building blocks of muscle tissue and play a role in satiety, helping you feel full longer. Including a good source of protein in your meal can also prevent muscle loss during the fasting period.

Carbohydrates have been demonized in many diet circles, but they're not the enemy. The key is choosing complex carbs—those found in whole grains, legumes, and starchy vegetables. They fuel your body with steady energy and provide critical fiber that can regulate digestion.

Fats used to be on the 'do not eat' list, but we now understand that healthy fats are vital. They're an energy source for your body and support the absorption of fat-soluble vitamins. Nuts, seeds, avocados, and olive oil are just a few examples of nutrient-rich fats that keep your body and brain powered up.

It's also time to focus on the micronutrients—vitamins and minerals. They may be needed in smaller quantities, but they're no less essential. Iron, calcium, and potassium are the unsung heroes that keep your bodily functions humming along gracefully.

Synchronizing your fiber intake with your fasting schedule can do wonders for your digestion and overall gut health. High-fiber foods like vegetables, fruits, and whole grains can aid in feeling full and ensuring smooth digestion during the eating window.

What about timing? The best strategy is to listen to your body. Some people thrive on eating their largest meal right after their fast, while others find a lighter meal works better. Tailoring your meal timing and size can help optimize your energy levels and prevent any digestive discomfort.

Planning is your ally. With a busy schedule, it's easy to find yourself hungry with no healthy options in sight. Meal prepping or having a set of go-tos can save you from making choices that steer you away from your fasting goals.

Lastly, don't forget to indulge every now and then. Yes, nourishment is critical, but so is enjoying your food. Allowing yourself an occasional treat can prevent feelings of deprivation and make fasting a genuinely balanced part of your life.

Remember, nutrition is the foundation of any successful fasting protocol. By focusing on eating for success, you'll support your body through the ebbs and flows of intermittent fasting, optimize your health, and set yourself up for sustainable progress. Here's to making informed, delightful choices at your next meal!

Essential Nutrients for Fasters

Embarking on a fasting journey requires not just a stout heart and a clear goal, but also a savvy approach to nourishing your body during your eating windows. This isn't a call to stockpile every vitamin on the shelf, but rather a suggestion to focus on essential nutrients that support your body's needs, particularly when it's in a fasting state.

Nutrients are the secret ingredients in your body's performance engine. Without them — think vitamins, minerals, and those fatty acids your body raves about — you'd be running on fumes. So, as you settle into an intermittent fasting schedule, your body's cry for wholesome nourishment should be heeded with the mindfulness of a Zen master. Let's dive into the nutritional goldmines you'll want to frequent.

Macro-must-haves, like proteins, are the heavy lifters. They're not just your muscle's best friend; they're also the architects of enzymes, hormones, and other body chemicals. When you're fasting, quality protein sources like lean meats, eggs, and legumes are vital to maintain muscle mass and keep your metabolism fiery.

Carbohydrates can be tricksters. They're the quick-burn fuel for energy, but it's the unrefined, complex carbs full of fiber that are the true gems. They'll keep digestion smooth and maintain blood sugar levels, which is something you'll cheer for during a fast. Spark up your diet with whole grains, vegetables, and fruits to snag these benefits.

Fats have been demonized, haven't they? But it's the types of fats that matter. Unsaturated fats — think avocados, nuts, and olive oil — are like silky priests bestowing blessings upon your heart health and cognitive function. Invest in them, store them, relish them. They're the kind of assets that pay dividends, especially when you're intermittently fasting and need sustainable energy sources.

Micronutrients might seem small, but their impact is massive. Vitamins and minerals are like the covert operatives working behind the scenes. Despite eating less frequently, you still need them in spades. Calcium and vitamin D are your bone's guardians, combating the briars of osteoporosis. Vegetables, dairy, and some fortified foods are where you'll find these treasures. For calcium, leafy greens like spinach and kale, and for vitamin D, the sun's greeting or, for the cave-dwellers among us, supplements and vitamin D-rich foods.

If there's a celebrity among vitamins for fasters, it's vitamin B12. When your meals are planned like a chess match, ensuring adequate B12 can feel like guarding your king. Vital for blood health and energy production, this vitamin is stashed in meat, fish, poultry, and dairy. Vegetarians and vegans? This is where supplements can step up to the plate.

Then there's the hydration hero, water. When fasting, you might be ditching meals, but you're not ditching water. In fact, let's highlight this—water is your ride or die. It keeps your physiological processes humming, flushes out the waste products of fat breakdown, and keeps energy levels steady.

Iron is another star, indispensable for energy levels and focus. Yet, it can be a slippery slope. Too little and you're fatigued; too much and you may invite trouble. Red meat, poultry, and fish are good sources, but for the plant-eaters, lentils, beans, and iron-fortified cereal with vitamin C-rich foods help your body absorb this precious metal.

Don't forget omega-3 fatty acids. Like a celebrity couple, they're stunning and powerful. Immune system support, anti-inflammatory properties, and brain health are their claim to fame. Fatty fish, walnuts, and flaxseeds will get you that omega-3 glow, and supplements are a solid backup dancer for those fish-free souls.

Zinc and magnesium are the unsung heroes. They're crucial for immune function, energy production, and even sleep - which, let me tell you, is an ally you want on your team when you're fasting. Seeds, nuts, whole grains, and dark leafy greens are the VIP lounges where these nutrients like to kick back.

Electrolytes — you've probably heard the term shouted from sports drink ads. However, it's not about chugging fluorescent-colored beverages. Balancing electrolytes like sodium, potassium, and magnesium is more nuanced when you're fasting. It's about moderated salt intake, reaching for an avocado or sweet potato for potassium, and maybe a dash of magnesium from a handful of almonds.

Now, I can almost hear the wheels turning in your mind, wondering about the timing of these nutrients. Just know, that precision isn't the goal; it's consistency and coverage throughout your feasting windows that count. It's like building a mosaic; piece by piece, the broader picture of your nutritional wellbeing forms.

Lastly, let's cast a spotlight on the mystical potion that is teas and herbal infusions. Your fasting hours needn't be stark and flavorless. Many tea varieties can offer subtle nutrition and benefits, from antioxidants to calming compounds, without breaking your fast. Consider them like the secret passages in haunted mansions - subtle but impactful.

Remember, the key to integrating essential nutrients into your fasting lifestyle isn't just about cramming them into your eating window; it's about weaving a tapestry of varied, nutrient-dense foods that support and enhance your fast, rather than detract from it. Keep it balanced, authentic, and above all, don't hesitate to consult with a nutritionist to tailor a plan that's as unique as you are. Your well-nourished fasting journey awaits!

Chapter 7

Fasting and Exercise

A Synergistic Approach

Stepping away from the nutritional components, it's time to dive into the dynamic duo of fasting and exercise, a game-changer in the world of health and fitness. The combination can seem daunting at first; after all, the common belief is that you need fuel to fire up those workouts. However, evidence suggests that when done correctly, aligning your exercise routine with your fasting schedule could actually ramp up your results. Let's explore how these two elements, when harmonized, can transform the efficiency of your body's energy utilization and bolster those weight loss efforts.

Picture this—your body, already a fat-burning machine from fasting, now has the added advantage of boosted metabolism from exercise. It doesn't just burn fat—it singes it! Exercise increases insulin sensitivity, which means that any food consumed post-workout is used more efficiently for recovery rather than just being stored as fat. Combined with the already enhanced insulin sensitivity from fasting, you're creating a prime environment for not just weight loss, but for improvements in overall health. It's like hitting two birds with one stone—except here, we're hitting fat and inefficiency with the might of fasting and exercise.

So, before you think about grabbing a snack pre-gym session, consider this: exercising in a fasted state encourages your body to pull from its fat reserves for energy. This won't just peak after one session. Over time, it trains your body to become more adept at fat utilization, which means you could potentially see quicker progress and more sustainable results. These sessions don't have to be marathons either—high-intensity interval training (HIIT), brisk walking, or even lifting weights can all integrate superbly with fasting to sculpt your body and sharpen your mind. In the upcoming pages, we'll dive into optimizing your workout performance and how to couple strength training with fasting without compromising muscle mass. For now, just know that this synergistic strategy could be your secret weapon against the weight loss plateau and toward achieving peak wellness.

Optimizing Workout Performance

Strike a balance—that's the mantra for merging fasting with your workout routine to supercharge both your health and your performance. It's an elegant dance between fueling the body and leaning into the periods of sustenance reprieve that unlocks a powerhouse of potential for those aiming to excel physically.

The notion of exercising in a fasted state has long been a subject of debate. Pitting an empty stomach against exercising might sound counterintuitive, and yet, it's a game-changer when done right. The secret here isn't just in the timing but in understanding the physiological symphony that is your metabolism.

Your body is adaptive, and cultivating this adaptability by incorporating fasting into your exercise regime can bolster your workout performance.

This doesn't mean plunging recklessly into a regime; rather, it necessitates a nuanced approach, one that centers on listening to your body's cues and responding with intelligent strategies.

Exercise, meet glycogen. When you tap into your fasting state, your body goes on a quest for energy, and in doing so, it scavenges from the surplus stored as glycogen in your muscles and liver. This forced frugality is beneficial—it teaches your cells to use fuel efficiently, promoting enhanced endurance and stamina.

What's equally captivating is how fasting can fine-tune your fat oxidation. Exercising on an empty tank encourages your body to torch fat for fuel. Picture this—those stubborn fat reserves you've been eyeing suspiciously? They're now front and center on the metabolic stage, being converted into useful energy, which translates to improved body composition over time.

Let's talk about growth hormone, a vital player in muscle health and recovery. Fasting induces spikes in growth hormone levels, which can lead to more significant muscle gains and quicker recovery. Add to that the reduction in inflammation, another fasting byproduct, and you're on track for fewer aches and speedy bounce-backs post-workout.

Now, this isn't a one-size-fits-all kind of deal. Men and women, young and seasoned athletes, can all harness the power of fasted workouts, but the devil is in the details. Timing and intensity are pivot points here—establishing a pre-workout fasting window that aligns with your daily rhythm can impact your energy levels and performance peaks.

The mind also plays a pivotal role. Mental toughness is forged in the fasting fires. Exercising while your body is in a fasted state requires a resolve that extends beyond physical capabilities—it's mental resilience that keeps you going when your energy stores wave the white flag.

Let's not dismiss the nutritional aspect. While fasting plays a leading role, replenishment after exercise is still crucial. Strategic refeeding post-workout with protein-rich and nutrient-dense foods facilitates muscle repair and growth, preventing catabolic breakdown.

Hydration is another cornerstone—fasting or not, water is essential, especially when you're demanding peak performance from your body. Keep the fluids flowing to ensure that you remain in tip-top shape both during and after your workouts.

We must caution against overreach, though. Rigorous exercise on a marathon fast? Ill-advised. Remember, fasting is a stressor on the body, much like exercise. When you couple the two, it magnifies their effects. Wisdom is in recognizing when to push and when to rest, when to challenge and when to nourish.

Variety is the spice of life, and it applies to your workouts, too. A medley of cardiovascular exercises and resistance training during different fasting states can elicit varied physiological benefits, accelerating your progress. Mixing it up keeps your body guessing, enhancing its adaptability and resilience.

Suppose you're looking to amplify your workout performance; consider the synergetic power of fasting as a launchpad. Every body is unique, and as with any change in diet or exercise, the golden rule is to check in with your healthcare provider.

To conclude, optimizing your workout performance with fasting is far from a mystical secret. It's vested in science, a touch of art, and a sprinkling of self-awareness. Whether it's summoning the endurance of a marathon runner or the brute strength of a powerlifter, fasting can be the wind beneath your wings—but it requires careful navigation. Pay attention to your body, prioritize recovery, and nourish smartly. That's the trifecta for unleashing your full potential.

As we progress, we'll delve deeper into how combining strength training and fasting can catalyze a transformation in your physical prowess. For now, let's revel in the knowledge that fasting, approached with mindfulness, isn't just about weight loss. It's about elevating every aspect of your wellbeing, and yes, that includes making you a force to be reckoned with, in the gym and beyond.

Combining Strength and Fasting

If you're deep into your exploration of fasting and exercise, you might be pondering a pivotal question: how does fasting fit into the puzzle of strength training? It's a great query. Fasting isn't just about endurance; it has a fascinating role in strength training. Let's peel back the layers on that association.

Many have the misconception that to build muscle, one must constantly fuel their body. However, fasting brings a new dimension to muscle development and strength gains. When you fast, your body undergoes hormonal adaptations which can enhance muscle growth and strength.

First, consider how fasting elevates growth hormone levels. This hormone aids in both fat loss and muscle gain. When in a fasted state, your body's natural growth hormone production increases, potentially leading to greater strength gains when you hit the weights.

Moreover, fasting can lead to increased insulin sensitivity. This means that when you do eat, your body can shuttle nutrients into muscle cells more efficiently, promoting muscle recovery and growth. It's not about eating more, but rather making what you eat work harder for you.

But what about energy? Surely, you need a steady stream of calories for those heavy lifting sessions? Here's where the body's adaptive nature shines. Fasting teaches your body to become more efficient at utilizing stored fat for energy, preserving muscle glycogen for when it's truly needed — like during a heavy squat or deadlift.

Of course, timing is critical. Aligning your eating windows with your strength training sessions can maximize nutrient uptake and muscle repair. It's like syncing two powerful forces — fasting and feeding — to work in concert for your strength-building goals.

Remember, strength training isn't merely about exerting force. It's also about recovery. Fasting may give your body the break it needs to focus on repairing and building muscle tissue. Without the constant task of digestion, the body can shift more resources to recovery.

There's also the aspect of mental toughness. Fasting builds a resilience that transcends the physical. The discipline required to abstain from eating can fortify your mental game, enhancing focus and grit during strength workouts.

Furthermore, don't overlook the benefit of reduced inflammation. Regular fasting can decrease inflammation in the body, promoting faster recovery and better overall health. This can be a boon for anyone looking to stay consistent with their strength training routine.

What about those who are skeptical or concerned about muscle catabolism? It's a common fear: the idea that fasting will cause the body to break down muscle for energy. However, muscle catabolism is less of a concern when fasting is combined with adequate protein intake and structured strength training. The body is smarter than we give it credit for; it prefers to burn fat over muscle when given the right conditions.

That said, it's not a one-size-fits-all approach. Personal experimentation is key. Some may thrive on shorter fasts, while others find their strength soars with longer periods of fasting. It's about finding that sweet spot where your body performs at its peak while still reaping the benefits of fasting.

To ease into combining strength training with fasting, start with less demanding sessions to gauge how your body responds. Gradually increase intensity as your body adapts. It's a learning process, but one that could pay off with impressive strength gains.

It's also important to consume nutrient-dense foods when you do eat. Maximizing your intake of vitamins, minerals, and amino acids can ensure your body has what it needs to build muscle and recover from workouts.

Lastly, staying hydrated is non-negotiable. Fasting or not, water plays a critical role in every bodily function, including muscle contraction and joint health. Ensure you're drinking plenty of fluids, especially around your training sessions.

In conclusion, when you marry the practice of fasting with strength training, you open up a world of possibilities for body composition and health. It's not just about lifting weights or skipping meals; it's about harmonizing these elements to create a stronger, more resilient body. The synergy of fasting and strength training awaits, potentially unlocking a potent pathway to achieving your fitness aspirations.

Chapter 8

Hormonal Harmony and Fasting

As we delve deeper into our journey of understanding the connection between intermittent fasting and weight loss, we touch upon a vital element often overlooked in traditional diet plans: hormonal harmony. The hormonal responses in our bodies are not just intricate—they're downright pivotal in determining how effectively we can manage our weight. Intermittent fasting isn't just about cutting calories; it's a strategic approach that aligns with our body's natural hormonal rhythms, supporting them to work for us rather than against us.

Now, let's center our focus on the main conductor of our body's hormonal orchestra: insulin. This hormone, essential for blood sugar regulation, can become out of tune due to constant eating and poor dietary choices, leading to insulin resistance—a culprit in weight gain and a host of health issues. Fasting acts as the balancing act, giving our bodies the necessary break from insulin spikes. This pause, in turn, increases insulin sensitivity, meaning less insulin is needed over time, encouraging our bodies to tap into stored fat for energy. Imagine this as fine-tuning a musical instrument, creating a melody that promotes a leaner physique and improved overall health.

But insulin isn't the only hormone affected by fasting. Let's not ignore the choir of other hormones like ghrelin, the hunger hormone, which finds a new, more subdued baseline, or leptin, which signals satiety and can start to send clearer messages after periods of fasting. Our endocrine system, responsible for hormone production, thrives on the ebb and flow that fasting brings about, crafting a symphony of hormonal balance that supports our wellbeing. Instead of a cacophony of cravings and energy crashes dictated by hormonal havoc, fasting introduces a rhythm where each hormone plays its part harmoniously, leading us towards achieving the elusive goal of sustainable weight loss.

Insulin Sensitivity and Regulation

So we've been exploring the broad strokes of how intermittent fasting can tip the scales in our favor—literally and figuratively. Now, let's delve into the nitty-gritty of why traditional dieting takes a back seat when it comes to the powerful duo of insulin sensitivity and regulation. It's a game where hormones call the shots, and insulin is your body's star quarterback.

Seeing as insulin is the traffic cop for glucose in our bloodstream, directing it to either be used as fuel or stored for later, it's pretty clear that this hormone needs to be working efficiently for optimal health. But let's be real—many of our lifestyles have thrown a wrench in insulin's ability to do its job effectively. The result? Decreased insulin sensitivity and the looming specter of various metabolic disorders.

Enter the stage: intermittent fasting. Think of fasting as that meticulous coach that helps insulin get its groove back. By periodically abstaining from food, you're not just giving your digestive system a break; you're signing up for an internal reset, training your body to respond to insulin more effectively. Because fasting can mean less frequent insulin spikes throughout the day, the sensitivity of your cells to this hormone can improve—a huge win.

Now, you might be thinking, "Insulin sensitivity sounds great and all, but what's it got to do with my waistline or health?" Plenty! When your cells listen and respond better to insulin, it means they're also better at managing glucose. Meaning, you could be looking at losing fat, stabilizing blood sugars, and even saying goodbye to that dreaded afternoon slump.

It's not just about reducing the amount of insulin in the game, though. The timing of when insulin enters the field is equally critical. By fasting, we orchestrate a dance where insulin makes fewer but more meaningful appearances, and we spare ourselves the chaos of constant insulin peaks and troughs. Stabilizing this hormonal rhythm can help manage appetite, reduce cravings, and lead to better food decisions when it is time to eat.

Some might say that frequent eating keeps the metabolic fires burning, but that's not necessarily the case. Frequent eating can keep insulin levels perpetually high, and over time, our cells can start to tune out its signal—a condition known as insulin resistance. This resistance prompts the pancreas to pump out even more insulin, and sooner or later, you're stuck in a loop that can be tough to escape.

Intermittent fasting challenges this cycle directly. It allows for periods where insulin can take a breather, providing time for insulin levels to naturally decline. This respite is like hitting a reset button, sensitizing your cells to insulin's call to action once more. It's all about balance, letting insulin do its job without overworking it.

Here's the kicker, though: all fasts are not created equal when it comes to insulin regulation. The length of your fast plays a crucial role. Shorter fasts might help get the ball rolling, but longer fasting periods might be where the true magic happens—a possibility worthy of exploration.

And this is not just about cutting back on the sugar or carbs, which, admittedly, is a part of the equation. This is about fundamentally changing the way our bodies deal with energy storage and usage. It goes deeper than just first-blush weight loss; it's about tweaking the very metabolism of our bodies for a long-term difference.

That said, it's critical to mention that fasting is a tool, not a cure-all. It's like exercise for your metabolism; it takes consistent effort, and it's not always a walk in the park. But by the same token, it comes with meaningful benefits that can extend beyond dropping pounds and can genuinely improve your metabolic health.

But hold on, let's not get too ahead of ourselves. We're not advocating for a free-for-all during eating windows. Quality of food matters, folks. The foods you choose can either support or hinder your journey toward increased insulin sensitivity. Whole foods, packed with nutrients, fiber, and without added sugars, tend to be the best teammates for insulin on this journey.

As you're navigating this road toward hormonal harmony, it's also essential to keep a close eye on how your body is responding. Some individuals may need a gentler approach to fasting or different timescales due to unique metabolic needs or health concerns. Patience and personalization are the name of the game for successful insulin regulation via fasting.

The bottom line is this: our bodies evolved with periods of feast and famine, and it's this natural cycling that can help keep our insulin regulation in check. It's about retraining our bodies to do what they do best—maintain a balance that supports our health and wellbeing. And intermittent fasting could be your ticket to getting back to that sweet spot where everything hums along just right.

So, as we gear up to integrate fasting into our lives, remember that each step toward better insulin sensitivity is a step toward a healthier, more vibrant you. The impact of fasting on hormonal regulation is profound, and with it comes a potential ripple effect of health benefits that could last a lifetime. It's time for a metabolic makeover, wouldn't you say?

The Impact on Other Hormones

While we've touched on the transformative effects of fasting on insulin levels, it's important to understand that the hormonal response to fasting is not limited to this single player on the field. In fact, it's a little like pulling one thread in a tapestry; pulling that insulin thread can cause a cascade of changes that run through the whole hormonal system. Let's unravel some more of this intricate hormonal tapestry together.

Begin with the stress hormones: cortisol and adrenaline. Now, these guys often get a bad rap, and sure, in chronic high levels, they're not exactly your best friends. However, in the context of intermittent fasting, stress hormones play an intriguing role. In the short term, they can actually increase your energy and focus—not what you might expect from a supposedly depleting fasting state. They are, in essence, part of your body's natural alertness mechanism, kind of like your biological cheerleaders, keeping you on your toes when food isn't coming in regularly.

Another hormonal tag team we can't ignore is the growth hormone (GH) and insulin-like growth factor 1 (IGF-1). Fasting has been shown to cause a significant surge in GH, which aids in fat loss and muscle preservation. It's like your own personal renovation project, breaking down the old, less efficient cells and building up the new. This pairs well with the decrease in IGF-1, which, although important for growth, may play a role in aging when constantly elevated. Fasting, then, becomes a powerful balancing act for these growth regulators.

Thyroid hormones also enter this complex dance. These hormones regulate metabolism, among other things, and fasting can initially create slight shifts in their levels. But before you worry about the metabolism slowing down, it's worth noting that these minor fluctuations are often temporary. As your body adapts to intermittent fasting, thyroid function often normalizes, reflecting the body's remarkable ability to maintain equilibrium.

Then there's leptin and ghrelin, the Yin and Yang of hunger hormones. Leptin tells you to put the fork down, while ghrelin is the one nudging you towards the snack cupboard. Intermittent fasting has the potential to sensitize the body's response to leptin, making it more attuned to satiety signals, which means you might feel full with less food. On the flip side, though ghrelin may spike initially, your body gradually adapts, and those hunger cues become less insistent, less often. It's like they're learning to take a hint that the kitchen's closed for a while.

And let's not forget about our mood and sex hormones like serotonin, dopamine, estrogen, and testosterone. Fasting affects these as well, and while the research is still evolving, the effects can be significant. For instance, the enhancement in mood due to elevated serotonin and dopamine levels during a fast might just surprise you with a feel-good buzz. As for estrogen and testosterone, balancing these hormones through fasting can have implications for everything from mood to muscle strength to libido.

With testosterone, men might find fasting particularly appealing. This hormone, vital for muscle development and overall vigor, tends to see a boost with regular fasting. On the other hand, women should be mindful as fasting can affect menstrual cycles and overall estrogen balance. Yet, when done thoughtfully, it can provide a platform for hormonal stabilization, showing how adaptable and responsive our body systems really are.

What stands out in this hormonal symphony is the undeniable interconnectedness. Hormones don't act in isolation; a change in one often reflects changes in others. It's a meticulous hormonal harmony that can be both fragile and resilient. Fasting is like a conductor's baton, initiating a subtle, yet profound orchestration of hormonal changes that can promote balance and health.

In this hormonal concert, the melody might seem complex at first, with high notes of increased stress hormones and low tones of shifting thyroid patterns. But as you fast regularly, the rhythm finds its groove, and the body fine-tunes the production and sensitivity of these hormones. This can contribute to not just weight loss, but also to overall wellbeing, energy levels, and even longevity. Who knew that skipping a meal could lead to such a profound systemic serenade?

We also have to consider the cumulative effects of all these hormonal shifts. It's not just about the peaks during fasting; it's about how these hormones level out and create a new balance post-fast. The body's natural rhythm starts to align with your fasting schedule, and over time, hormonal responses that once seemed like massive fluctuations begin to stabilize, fostering a more harmonious hormonal environment.

Of course, every person's hormonal response is as unique as their finger-print, influenced by genetics, lifestyle, stress levels, and overall health. This individual variability means that the fasting journey and its hormonal out-comes will differ from person to person. One individual may experience significant changes in their hunger hormones, while another might find their mood or energy levels are the most markedly improved.

Bearing in mind this individuality, it's crucial to approach fasting with a spirit of curiosity and self-observation. Monitoring how your body and mood respond as you delve into fasting can provide valuable insights, enabling you to tailor your fasting approach to suit your unique hormonal landscape. Listening to your body's signals is key—it's almost as if your hormones are trying to tell you a story, and it's your job to listen.

In the end, fasting is not just about weight loss; it's about learning to live in harmony with your body's natural processes. Hormones are the chem-ical messengers that help orchestrate these processes, and understanding their role can be the difference between struggling with your weight and achieving true, sustainable wellbeing. Intermittent fasting isn't just a diet; it's a path to hormonal balance and, in turn, a healthier, more vibrant life.

So, as we continue to peel back the layers of how intermittent fasting in-fluences our body, one thing is becoming abundantly clear: the impact on our hormone health is profound and far-reaching. The benefits of fasting extend beyond the simple caloric deficits of traditional diets, tapping into the body's inherent wisdom, and unlocking its full potential. It's not just about what we eat or when we eat; it's about how our bodies respond, adapt, and ultimately thrive.

Now that we've explored the delicate interplay of hormones affected by fasting, you're likely equipped with a new lens through which to view your health and weight loss goals. Harnessing the power of fasting to optimize these hormonal interactions can be transformative, setting the stage for success where other diets fall short. A balanced hormonal milieu is within reach—and it could be just a fast away.

Chapter 9

Fasting for Women
Special Considerations

When exploring the world of intermittent fasting, we come across a landscape rich with benefits, physiological changes, and empowering resets. However, stepping into this terrain requires us to recognize that men and women can experience fasting quite differently. It isn't a one-size-fits-all approach—especially for women. The female body orchestrates a complex ballet of hormones, each with specific roles. This delicate dance is essential to a woman's wellbeing and reproductive health, and fasting can impact this choreography in distinct ways. So, let's dive into the nuances of fasting for women and unearth the specific considerations that need to be accounted for to maintain health and achieve the best results.

Ladies, have you ever noticed how your energy levels, appetite, and mood seem to be in flux over the course of the month? These variations are tied to the ebb and flow of your hormonal cycles. Fasting inadvertently steps onto this hormonal stage—and it's crucial to understand its effects. For example, the luteal phase of your menstrual cycle, the phase post-ovulation, is a time when your body is more sensitive to stress. A prolonged fast during this period might exacerbate feelings of fatigue or irritability. By tuning into these signals, women can tailor their fasting schedules to align harmoniously with their hormonal rhythms, empowering them to optimize their fasting experience.

However, there are stages in a woman's life—such as pregnancy and menopause—where the body undergoes profound shifts that must be honored. Pregnancy is a time of heightened nutritional demand, not just for sustaining the mother but also for supporting the growth and development of the baby. Fasting during pregnancy is commonly advised against, as it can interfere with these crucial developmental stages. Menopause, on the other hand, represents another significant hormonal shift, with a new set of nutritional and metabolic considerations. A woman's body is seeking a new equilibrium during this transition, and fasting can be a tool to help mitigate some menopausal symptoms, but it's critical to approach it with gentleness and a deep understanding of one's own body signals. It's not about zealously adhering to a strict regimen—it's about learning to dance with your body's rhythms and fast in a way that supports rather than challenges your wellbeing.

Addressing Hormonal Fluctuations

As we dive deeper into the topic of fasting, especially for women, we can't overlook the intricate dance of hormonal fluctuations. Women experience unique hormonal changes that can significantly impact their fasting experience and metabolic outcomes. Understanding these nuances helps carve out a fasting plan that is harmonious with a woman's physiological makeup.

First up, let's discuss the monthly cycle. A woman's menstrual cycle is orchestrated by a complex interplay of hormones like estrogen and progesterone, which can affect hunger, energy, and mood. These hormones follow a rhythm of their own, and fasting may influence their levels, and vice versa. It's not uncommon for women to notice shifts in their fast tolerance during different phases of their cycle.

During the follicular phase, which is the first half of the menstrual cycle, estrogen is on the rise. This hormone is associated with higher energy levels, and some women may find it more comfortable to fast during this time. On the flip side, appetite can increase just before ovulation. Women might want to listen to their bodies and ease up on fasting intensity around this time.

Heading into the luteal phase, things can get a bit trickier. After ovulation, if pregnancy does not occur, progesterone rises, potentially increasing appetite and cravings, especially for carbs. This doesn't mean fasting is off the table, but adaptation might be necessary. Shortening fasting windows or allowing for more flexible eating patterns here can support a woman's hormonal health.

Then, for those entering perimenopause or menopause, a whole different hormonal shift occurs. Declining estrogen levels are the hallmark of this transition and can come with a suite of challenges, from hot flashes to disrupted sleep, which can affect fasting practices.

Embracing fasting around these transitions may require an increased emphasis on nutrient density during eating periods. It is also helpful to maintain a consistent eating schedule to help mitigate the stress on the body that fluctuating hormones already cause.

Adrenal health plays a significant role in coping with hormonal ebbs and flows during fasting. The adrenals produce stress hormones like cortisol, which can be increased due to fasting stress, especially in women. If cortisol levels rise too high for too long, it can preempt weight loss and lead to other health issues. That's why incorporating relaxation techniques and ensuring sufficient sleep during fasting regimens is crucial.

Thyroid hormones should also be on the radar when discussing fasting and female hormonal health. The thyroid, responsible for regulating metabolism, can be sensitive to dietary changes, including calorie restriction or fasting. Women, in particular, are more prone to thyroid disorders. A balanced approach to fasting, avoiding overly prolonged fasts, can help safeguard thyroid function.

For women with polycystic ovary syndrome (PCOS), fasting might offer some benefits, as it can help improve insulin sensitivity, a common concern with PCOS. But again, the keyword here is balance. A well-thought-out fasting plan that does not exacerbate stress on the body is essential to avoid hormonal imbalances.

Let's not forget about the hormone leptin, which signals fullness, and its counterpart, ghrelin, which signals hunger. These hormones, too, can be affected by fasting. Women may experience spikes in ghrelin during fasting periods, making it harder to continue the fast. Monitoring hunger signals and tailoring the fasting approach can aid in managing these hormonal signals effectively.

When considering long-term fasting, reproductive hormones must be considered. Extended periods of intense caloric restriction can lead to irregular menstrual cycles or amenorrhea, the absence of menstruation. This is not just a nuisance but can also affect bone health and fertility. Therefore, adopting a fasting rhythm that respects the body's need for nourishment and reproductive function is paramount.

It's also worth mentioning that fasting can be a double-edged sword regarding mood and cognitive function due to hormonal interplay. While some women report heightened clarity and energy, others might experience mood swings or brain fog. Honing in on this personal experience empowers women to adapt their fasting routines for their wellbeing.

In conclusion, while fasting holds tremendous potential for health and weight management, women need to consider their unique hormonal landscape when crafting their fasting schedules. Equipped with this knowledge, women can optimize their fasts without disrupting the delicate hormonal balance that underpins their overall health and wellbeing.

Lastly, integration and patience are vital. Hormones do not adjust overnight, nor should the fasting plan be rigid. A gentle, mindful approach that evolves with a woman's changing body ensures that fasting remains a sustainable and beneficial part of her wellness repertoire.

Maintaining dialogue with healthcare providers, staying in tune with one's body, and adjusting fasting patterns in response to hormonal cues are key. In the upcoming sections, we'll delve into specific circumstances like Pregnancy and Menopause, and how to adapt fasting strategies accordingly. But for now, let's remember that fasting isn't one-size-fits-all—especially for women—and that adjusting our sails to the winds of hormonal change is not just smart; it's essential for lasting success.

Pregnancy, Menopause, and Fasting

When it comes to women's health, few things are as complex or as beautiful as the cycles of life that include pregnancy and menopause. Both are significant phases that come with their own challenges and considerations, especially when we introduce fasting into the mix. It's essential to navigate these waters with care, aware of the profound impacts our dietary choices can have during these times.

For women who are pregnant or looking to conceive, the primary focus should always be on providing both the mother and the developing baby with enough nutrients for optimal health. During pregnancy, fasting isn't typically recommended as the baby's growth and development rely on a constant supply of nutrients from the mother. Moreover, the metabolic demands of pregnancy increase, requiring additional caloric intake. This doesn't mean that you should abandon all aspects of a regulated eating plan, but rather adapt it to fit these heightened nutritional needs.

As for women navigating the fluctuating hormone levels of perimenopause and menopause, fasting poses a different set of considerations. These life stages mark the end of the reproductive years and the onset of a new phase, where the body undergoes significant hormonal changes. These changes can have a range of effects, from weight gain to increased risk of certain diseases like osteoporosis and heart disease.

Now, let's delve into the world of fasting amidst these hormonal tidal waves. Some preliminary research tells us that fasting during menopause could, in fact, help manage some of the accompanying symptoms. This includes potential weight loss, improved insulin sensitivity, and even a sense of regained control during a time when so much feels in flux.

Weight gain, particularly around the abdomen, is a common concern as women transition into menopause. Fasting regimens have been shown to promote fat loss while preserving muscle mass – both of which are incredibly valuable during this stage of life. However, it's not just about shedding pounds; it's about respecting the body's changing needs and metabolism.

Bone health is another crucial factor for women, particularly post-menopause. Intermittent fasting might affect how the body metabolizes calcium and other vital nutrients for bone health, so if there's an already existing risk or a family history of osteoporosis, fasting may need to be implemented with extra caution, ensuring that nutrient intake remains adequate.

Another aspect of menopause is the change in sleep patterns and mood swings due to hormonal fluctuations. Fasting, when timed appropriately, can aid in regulating the sleep-wake cycle, potentially improving sleep quality. And let's not overlook the empowerment a woman can feel when she takes control of her eating patterns. This psychological boost can be a welcome side effect during an often challenging time.

It's essential to keep in mind that fasting during menopause isn't a one-size-fits-all fix. Each woman's experience of menopause is as unique as her fingerprint, and any fasting approach should be individually tailored. A less intensive fasting protocol might be more appropriate, focusing on shorter fasting periods and ensuring that fasting doesn't exacerbate symptoms like hot flashes or dip energy levels too low.

Throughout these life stages, keeping a close eye on nutrient density is important. For pregnant women who may still practice mild forms of time-restricted eating for health reasons, it's all about maximizing the nutritional bang for each bite. For menopausal women, a nutrient-rich diet paired with a reasonable fasting schedule can support the body's changing needs.

Listening to your body becomes increasingly important here. For both pregnant and menopausal women, if fasting induces stress or discomfort, it's a signal to reassess and adjust accordingly. Adequate hydration is crucial during fasting, but this is especially so for pregnant and menopausal women who may have different hydration needs.

Consulting with healthcare providers is indispensable. Whether you're considering fasting while pregnant or during menopause, professional guidance not only ensures safety but also provides a personalized approach that aligns with your body's specific requirements. Remember, each phase of a woman's life is unique, and so should her approach to fasting.

Moving beyond these life phases, the post-menopausal period can be an ideal time to embrace fasting more fully. With the reproductive years behind, women can often fast with a bit more flexibility, provided that they remain mindful of their overall health status. It's a time that can be viewed as a new beginning, one where fasting might be a robust tool for maintaining health and vitality.

So, whether you're navigating the seas of pregnancy or steering through the waves of menopause, fasting demands a tailored touch – a personalized tweak to accommodate and align with the hormonal ballet that orchestrates a woman's life. It shouldn't be a source of stress but a method by which you can reclaim a sense of agency over your health and wellbeing.

Remember, fasting isn't just about time spent without food; it's also about the quality of nourishment when you do eat. For women in these life stages, the focus should pivot not just to "when" but also to "what" and "how much." It's a holistic approach to health that honors the uniqueness of the female body during all its seasons.

In conclusion, applying fasting as a tool for health and wellness can be profoundly empowering for women, especially during pregnancy and menopause. With respect, awareness, and appropriate care, fasting can be integrated into a woman's life in a way that supports her wellbeing through these significant transitions. It's a dance with the natural rhythms of the body, a respectful partnership between fasting and femininity that, when choreographed thoughtfully, can lead to a symphony of health benefits. Embrace the journey, and let your body's innate wisdom guide you through these transformative phases of life with grace and strength.

Chapter 10

Managing Social and Lifestyle Factors

As we've seen, intermittent fasting offers a flexible approach to healthy living, but what happens when real life enters the mix? You know, that whirlwind of social outings, family dinners, and weekend getaways that make a strict regimen seem near impossible. Let's talk strategy. Navigating your social life while maintaining your fasting schedule isn't just doable; it's key for sustainable change. It's about adaptability—aligning your fasting windows with social events when you can and learning not to sweat it when life throws you a curveball. You're crafting a lifestyle, not shackling yourself to an inflexible system.

Hitting the road doesn't have to throw a wrench in your fasting goals, either. Travel, be it for work or play, often shakes up our daily routine. But rather than seeing this as a barrier, view it as an opportunity to practice intermittent fasting in a new environment. Whether it's adjusting your eating window to accommodate a different time zone or selecting healthier food choices while out and about, remember you're in the driver's seat. This isn't about perfection; it's about making better choices, step by step, meal by meal.

Consider this: intermittent fasting isn't a diet; it's a consolidation of meal timing that complements your lifestyle, not complicates it. So, as life's events unfold, remember that flexibility is your friend. Go out, enjoy that family barbecue, and embrace occasional indulgence as part of the journey. What's most important is returning to your fasting routine without guilt. After all, the beauty of this lifestyle lies in its simplicity and sustainability. It's about finding the balance that works for you, and keeping your eye on the long game—your health.

Navigating Social Settings

Navigating social settings while maintaining a fasting schedule can seem daunting at first. There's the peer pressure, the temptations of delicious food, and the fear of missing out at gatherings. However, with the right strategies and mindset, it's not only feasible but also relatively stress-free to stay true to your intermittent fasting plan while enjoying a vibrant social life.

Firstly, it's crucial to remember you're not alone. Many individuals are adopting intermittent fasting as a lifestyle. Often, you'll find that friends and family are supportive once they understand your goals. Moreover, having a robust support system can work wonders for your motivation and adherence to your fasting schedule.

It's vital to plan ahead when you know you'll be attending a social event. If it's scheduled during your eating window, that's great; you can enjoy your meal with everyone else. If it's not, consider shifting your fasting schedule slightly to accommodate it. Flexibility within reason is key to making your fasting plan work long-term.

Communication is your ally. Don't be shy to let the host know about your fasting. You don't need to delve into a deep scientific explanation, but a brief mention can prevent any awkwardness when you skip a meal or turn down an appetizer. It's about finding a balance between being sociable and being true to your health regimen.

Bring a fasting-friendly beverage, like sparkling water or herbal tea, to social events. Sipping on one of these can keep your hands busy and satisfy the urge to consume something without breaking your fast. It's also a subtle way to blend in with the eating and drinking happening around you.

Remember, intermittent fasting isn't a diet; it's a lifestyle adjustment. Being too rigid can lead to unnecessary stress. If you happen to break your fast earlier than planned, don't beat yourself up. Acknowledge the situation, enjoy the moment, and plan to get back on track with your next fasting window.

At restaurants, selecting fasting-friendly options can be a winning strategy. Opt for foods that align with your eating plan, and focus on portion control. It's all about making intelligent choices that mesh your social life with your health goals without causing too much friction or drawing undue attention to your eating habits.

If you're faced with an impromptu food situation, like an office birthday party or a spontaneous outing, a polite decline or choosing to participate minimally can be acceptable. You can always suggest a non-food related activity as an alternative way to celebrate or socialize.

Also, don't forget to enjoy the non-eating aspects of social gatherings. Dance, converse, and participate in games or whatever festivities are on offer. Socializing doesn't have to revolve around food and drinks, and you might find that fasting helps enhance your presence and enjoyment at these events.

When alcohol is involved, it can be a bit more complicated. If you choose to drink, do so responsibly and consider how it fits into your fasting window. Some choose to abstain completely during fasting periods or only partake lightly during their eating windows to avoid any potential disruption to their fasting goals.

For holidays and special occasions that are traditionally centered around meals, focus on the spirit of the celebration rather than the food. Share stories, laugh, and connect with loved ones. You can always enjoy a festive dish later during your designated eating times.

Let's also talk about peer pressure—it's real, and it can be a challenge. Having a few polite, go-to responses can help you navigate these situations gracefully. Often, a simple "Thanks, I'm good for now" or "I'm not hungry at the moment, but everything looks fantastic" will suffice.

If you're on a tighter fasting schedule, such as OMAD (One Meal A Day), it requires more strategic planning and perhaps a bit more explanation to curious friends. But remember, your health journey is personal, and it's okay to put your needs first.

Finally, consider starting a social group or finding a community centered around intermittent fasting. Online forums, local meetups, and group chats can provide additional support and advice on how to navigate the social aspects of fasting. Plus, sharing experiences and strategies for social settings can make sticking to your fasting plan easier.

In conclusion, integrating fasting into your social life isn't about sacrifice; it's about strategic adjustments and prioritizing your wellbeing while enjoying the richness of life's social tapestry. With the right approach, you can maintain your intermittent fasting lifestyle and still partake in the joy and connection that social events provide.

Traveling While Fasting

Embarking on a journey—whether it's a quick business trip or an extended vacation—doesn't mean you have to derail your intermittent fasting plan. In fact, it's possible to marry the spontaneity of travel with the discipline of fasting, weaving together an experience that's both liberating and aligned with your health goals. Let's navigate these potentially choppy waters and come out on the other side, triumphant and still on track.

First, consider your fasting schedule and how it can dovetail with your travel plans. If you're due to board a flight during your typical eating window, adjust your eating period ahead of time. Gradual shifts a few days prior can prevent an abrupt change that your body might not welcome. You're in control here, so tweak the timing to suit your itinerary—this isn't about fasting taking over your life; it's about making fasting fit comfortably within it.

Staying hydrated is key, especially when you're up in the air or traversing different climates. Water can be your pal through your fasting hours, but don't forget that you can add some life to it: a squeeze of lemon, a pinch of salt, or a dash of herbs for a bit of flavor. Coffee and tea are also on the table—just keep them unsweetened to prevent any insulin spikes that would break your fast.

Handling hunger pangs while traveling is as much about distraction as it is about determination. Have you ever noticed how being absorbed in a captivating activity causes you to forget about eating? Use this natural tendency to your advantage. Dive into a novel, strike up a conversation with a fellow traveler, or lose yourself in a podcast. By the time you resurface, you'll likely have sailed past the temptation to snack.

Dining out while fasting on the road might seem daunting, but it's more about making informed choices. Scope out eateries that offer fresh, whole foods that can fit into your eating window. Then, when it's time to dine, savor every bite without guilt—after all, this is as much a part of the travel experience as sightseeing is.

Time zone changes can complicate fasting schedules, but they're nothing you can't handle with a little planning. Sync your fasting to local times as swiftly as possible. This might mean you're fasting a bit longer one day or less the next, but consistency will quickly return once your body adjusts to the new schedule.

For longer trips, flexibility is your best friend. If your fasting plan becomes overwhelming, it's perfectly fine to ease up on the reins. Aiming for a shorter fasting period or shifting to alternate-day fasting can alleviate some of the stressors. Remember, the goal is sustainability—pushing yourself too hard could be counterproductive.

Tapping into local culture can enhance your travel experience and adherence to your fasting routine. Delving into local cuisine during your eating window can be a rewarding exploration that complements your fasting journey. This immersion can make fasting feel more like a part of the adventure rather than an obligation.

The occasional indulgence isn't just acceptable—it's human. If a once-in-a-lifetime foodie opportunity presents itself, it's okay to take a break from fasting. Enjoying these moments guilt-free and then returning to your routine afterward can reinforce a healthy relationship with both fasting and food.

Speaking of indulgence, it's important to be mindful of food quality during your eating windows. Fast food might be convenient, especially when you're on the move, but prioritizing nutritious meals will help maintain your energy levels and support your fasting efforts. Aim for balance: proteins, fibers, healthy fats—the good stuff that keeps you feeling full longer.

Concerned about jet lag? Fasting might actually help mitigate its effects. Some advocate for fasting during your flight and then breaking your fast with a meal timed to the local meal schedule. This not only anchors your body's new circadian rhythm but also gives your digestion a rest during transit.

Don't neglect the social component of traveling while fasting. If your travel companions aren't fasting, there's no need to isolate yourself during meal times. Join the table, engage in the conversation, and enjoy a sparkling water while others eat. You can still partake in the social experience, reinforcing that fasting doesn't have to mean sacrificing making memories.

If you're worried about staying on track, preparation goes a long way. Pack some fasting-friendly items for your journey—such as herbal teas, electrolyte packets, or even a small vial of apple cider vinegar to add to your water. Being equipped can help you ward off temptation and maintain your fasting momentum.

Last but not least, staying connected to your fasting community or support system while traveling can provide a much-needed boost. Share your experiences, your challenges, and even celebrate your wins. This camaraderie can be an invaluable source of both information and motivation.

To sum up, traveling while fasting might have its unique twists and turns, but with a dash of foresight and a sprinkle of flexibility, you can thrive. By staying mindful and planning ahead, you can embrace the joy of discovery on the road without losing sight of your intermittent fasting objectives. It's not about putting your life on pause—it's about enhancing the experience, one mindful decision at a time.

Chapter 11

Advanced Fasting Protocols

As we've navigated the ins and outs of intermittent fasting, it's clear that there's more to this journey than skipping breakfast or pushing back dinner. For those of you who've dipped your toes in the intermittent fasting pool and are now ready to dive deeper, advanced fasting protocols can offer a new plateau of benefits. Now, this isn't about testing your willpower to the extreme or pushing beyond your body's signals. Instead, advanced fasting is a sophisticated dance with time, one that harmonizes with our body's innate rhythm to unlock profound metabolic healing and cellular rejuvenation.

Imagine fasting as an orchestra, and you've been conducting the foundational pieces with mastery. It's time for the symphony to evolve, to introduce complexity with extended periods of fasting that invite your body to delve into its hidden reserves. By doing so carefully and intentionally, you coax your body into states where autophagy – the body's way of cleaning house at the cellular level – becomes more pronounced. While we've hinted at cellular cleanup in previous chapters, advanced protocols place a greater focus on this process, aiming to offer longevity and a robust shield against the ailments that the modern world throws our way.

To practice advanced fasting safely and effectively, we must approach it with the same respect as we would any powerful tool. It's crucial to move forward with a well-informed strategy, balancing our body's signals with our desired outcomes. By now, you understand the importance of tuning in to your body's cues. The same principle applies here, perhaps even more so. Just as a skillful artist knows when to add depth to their painting, you'll learn to recognize when your body is primed for a deeper fast, ensuring the process remains a rejuvenate rather than a deplete. Remember, this stage isn't for everyone, and that's perfectly fine. But for those ready to explore beyond the shores of conventional fasting schedules, advanced fasting protocols await to unlock a new dimension of health and vitality.

Extended Fasting Periods

Welcome to the world of extended fasting periods, where the real magic happens for those looking to deepen their fasting practice both for weight loss and for its numerous health benefits. Extended fasting – which typically refers to periods ranging from 24 hours to several days – is a step beyond intermittent fasting protocols you may already be familiar with. It's not something to be taken lightly or dived into without preparation, but with the right knowledge and approach, it can be a game-changer.

First, let's talk about what happens to your body during an extended fast. After the 24-hour mark, you're likely to find that your body has shifted into a state of ketosis. This means that, having used up its glucose stores, it's now turning to fat for fuel. It's a metabolic transition that comes with a noticeable surge in energy for many, and it's also where you'll start to notice significant weight loss benefits.

Aside from the clear metabolic shift, there are mental and emotional benefits to be mined from these longer periods without food. Many fasters report a sense of mental clarity and heightened alertness - that fog you didn't even know was there lifts, and you can suddenly take on the world. Extended fasting can be a mental reset as much as a physical one.

A crucial part of embarking on these extended fasting periods is ensuring your body is ready. Preferably, you're already accustomed to shorter fasts and have a baseline of health that supports going without food for longer stretches. Safety should always be your priority, so it's also wise to consult with a healthcare professional before starting such a regimen.

As you go beyond the 24-hour mark, you might be wondering about things like 'starvation mode' - a misused term that's often incorrectly thrown into the conversation about fasting. What actually happens during extended fasting is quite beneficial: your body becomes incredibly efficient at utilizing its stores, and contrary to slowing down, your metabolism can actually increase in the short term.

One of the greatest draws to extended fasting is the potential for autophagy, a process we'll discuss in more depth later, but just know that this is your body's power cleanse. When you're not loading it up with food to process, it turns its attention to cleaning house, repairing cells, and getting rid of anything that doesn't serve your health.

Now, navigating the world of extended fasting means listening to your body. If at any point you feel unwell beyond the expected hunger pangs, it's time to reassess. Hydration is key, and you'll want to ensure you're getting enough minerals and electrolytes. Experts often recommend bone broth or electrolyte supplements for this very reason.

The talk of electrolytes brings us neatly to a common concern: How do you maintain proper nutrition while not consuming food? The answer lies in strategic supplementation and a well-planned refeeding process after the fast. When you do eat, you should focus on nutrient-dense foods that support your body's recovery and continued health.

A note on the psychological front: extended fasting is as much a mental challenge as a physical one. It can be a battle of wills with that part of your mind that's used to grabbing a snack whenever the slightest hunger cue appears. Approaching extended fasts with mindfulness and a clear understanding of why you're doing it can provide the mental strength required to see it through.

Of course, extended fasting isn't suitable for everyone. Specific populations, including pregnant women, people with a history of eating disorders, and those with certain medical conditions, should avoid it. It's a powerful tool but must be respected as such.

For those ready to embrace extended fasting, preparation is the golden ticket. Some find it helpful to gradually increase the length of their fasting windows over time. Others jump in a little more quickly but take extra care to listen to their bodies and stop if needed. There's no one-size-fits-all approach; it's about finding what works for you.

Refeeding after an extended fast is an art in itself. The key is to not overwhelm the digestive system. Starting with small portions of easily digestible foods and gradually increasing intake will allow your body to adapt without distress. This cautious approach will help maintain the benefits of your fast without causing undue strain on your system.

Lastly, it's important to recognize that extended fasting can affect people differently. The experience is subjective, and while one person may feel euphoric and full of energy after 48 hours, another may feel the need to break the fast sooner. It's about personal limits and respecting your body's signals.

In summary, extended fasting holds profound potential for those seeking to enhance their health and change their relationship with food. It's a step up from the intermittent fasting patterns you're used to, requiring preparation, patience, and respect for your body's capabilities and limits. But for those who step up to the challenge, it could well be the key to unlocking a more vibrant, healthful life.

Autophagy and Cellular Cleaning

As we delve into the art of fasting, we uncover powerful processes beyond the simple reduction of waistline numbers. Yes, fasting can shrink your body fat, but it can also awaken a mighty cellular janitor—autophagy. This sophisticated process is the unsung hero of cellular maintenance, a form of internal decluttering that trashes the old, worn-out cellular components and helps in regenerating newer, healthier ones.

To give you a peek into this microscopic world—think of your cells as bustling cities. Just like urban landscapes, cells accumulate waste and debris. The build-up of such cellular residue can contribute to aging and diseases. That's where autophagy, which literally translates to "self-eating," steps in. During fasting, when the constant influx of external nutrients halts, your cells turn inward for energy. It is as if they start to 'clean house' by breaking down and recycling their own parts.

But why should we care about this inner cellular cleanse? Because the implications for health and longevity are staggering. Autophagy helps combat the onset of neurodegenerative diseases, bolsters the immune system, and couples with anti-inflammatory effects to create an all-around health elixir that medicine cannot match.

The relationship between fasting and autophagy is akin to sleep and rest—essential, restorative, and quite frankly, non-negotiable. Extending your fasting periods pushes your cells into deeper levels of autophagy. Here's the clincher: It's like pressing a reset button on your body. It's how your cells can purge the junk that could be the precursor to a myriad of health issues.

So, how do you ignite this powerful cellular process? It's not as easy as flipping a switch; it's about fasting duration. Short-term fasts might not be enough to fully kick-start autophagy. Researchers suggest that it often requires fasting for longer periods—somewhere around the 16-hour mark, with more profound effects noted as the fasting time increases.

Imagine your cells as little factories. During a fast, these factories switch from production mode to maintenance mode. They start to pick through parts, selecting the malfunctioning pieces and converting them into energy. It's a recycling system that not only benefits cellular health but also conserves energy resources. It's the ultimate in efficiency—ideal for a society that's increasingly environmentally conscious, right?

Let's not forget that autophagy plays a pivotal role in preventing the accumulation of damaged proteins linked to several diseases. Think about conditions like Alzheimer's and other related cognitive decline issues. Autophagy is critical here. By clearing out potentially harmful protein aggregates, it's like putting up a barrier to protect against these debilitating conditions.

Now, fasting for autophagy isn't just about randomly going without food. There's a finesse to it. The intensity and timing matter. Just as a well-oiled machine runs on specific schedules and parameters, your body requires a degree of precision when engaging in fasting protocols to optimize autophagy.

But patience is essential. The biological symphony of autophagy doesn't play out instantaneously. As you ease into longer fasting periods, your body slowly adapts, and autophagy rates tend to increase. It's like training for a marathon—progress unfolds over time. As you become more accustomed to fasting, you allow your cells the luxury of time to meticulously clean and repair themselves.

A potential game-changer in the war against age-related decline, autophagy not only gives cells a new lease on life but also appears to rejuvenate the entire immune system. It's as if every fast triggers a spark that rejuvenates the body's defenses. With a stronger shield against pathogens, you're not just leaner—you're more resilient.

Bear in mind, that autophagy isn't an exclusively fasting-induced phenomenon. Certain nutrients and compounds can also influence it, albeit not as powerfully as fasting does. Yet, when these nutrients align with your fasting regimen, they may act like an assistive force, nudging autophagy along its path. It's worth mentioning, though, not to rely solely on supplements to do the heavy lifting—fasting is the key driver here.

While the mechanisms may sound complex, the message is clear: Fasting translates into profound cellular cleansing that impacts your vitality on a scale that's almost poetic. Autophagy isn't just cleaning up cellular waste; it's about giving your body the chance to reset and thrive. It redefines what it means to cleanse your body, extending beyond the surface into the molecular dance of life and death within your cells.

Embracing advanced fasting protocols intending to activate autophagy requires respect for your body's cues and understanding the nuanced responses it gives during an extended fast. It's a dialogue with yourself, where listening is as important as the act of fasting itself. With time and practice, you grow attuned to the signals your body sends and learn how best to support the natural cycles of renewal through fasting-induced autophagy.

In conclusion, while fasting strips away the extra pounds, autophagy sweeps away the cellular debris, setting the stage for a healthier, more vibrant you. As your body cleanses itself from the inside out, you may find that fasting transcends weight loss, elevating your well-being on a fundamental level. It's a testament to the power of taking a step back from the constant onslaught of eating, offering your body the chance to do what it does best—nurture and repair itself through the magic of autophagy.

Chapter 12

Common Questions and Troubleshooting

As you've journeyed through the science, psychology, and social dance of intermittent fasting, you've no doubt encountered some bumps along the way—challenges that can make even the most resolute faster question their path. This chapter is designed like a trusty pocket guide, ready to unfold the solutions to common hurdles and answer the burning questions that can arise during your fasting journey. It's normal to hit snags, whether it's grappling with hunger pangs that seem to echo through your being or navigating through those pesky weight plateaus that test your resolve.

Let's cut through the noise—troubleshooting is part and parcel of any lifestyle change, particularly one that involves rewriting your body's rulebook on eating. One of the most inescapable questions is how to effectively manage hunger and cravings without resorting to a feeding frenzy. We'll delve into practical, grounded strategies that you can tailor to your hunger cues, nutritional needs, and even the most impulsive cravings. Whether it's leveraging the power of hydrating strategies, understanding the satiety equation, or smart snacking—yes, it can fit into your intermittent fasting plan—you'll gather the tools needed to stay on track without feeling deprived.

Now, what about those times when it feels like your progress is stuck in molasses—those dreaded plateaus? We understand the frustration, but there's good news—plateaus are both common and surmountable. They're a sign your body is adapting, so consider them a challenge to outsmart rather than an impassable wall. We will explore strategies to reignite your metabolic engine and potentially tweak your fasting protocol. Adjusting your plan isn't a setback; it's a sign of progress. Embracing flexibility and patience can help you to optimize your fasting routine and push beyond the standstill. With the collected wisdom in this chapter, you'll be ready to tackle the common questions and keep your fasting journey on a steady, upward trajectory.

Handling Hunger and Cravings

Hunger and cravings can be the Achilles' heel for anyone embarking on a journey of intermittent fasting. It's both a mental and physical challenge that often leads to the question, "How can one keep these at bay without giving in?" This section is dedicated to deconstructing that obstacle and equipping you with strategies to overcome it effectively.

Let's start with understanding hunger. Fundamentally, hunger is your body's natural signal that it needs energy. However, cravings are more complex; they're shaped by emotional state, environment, and, often, habit. The good news is that intermittent fasting teaches you to differentiate between true hunger and mere desire for food.

Initially, hunger pangs may feel more pronounced, but there's light at the end of the tunnel. As your body adapts to fasting, it becomes more efficient at utilizing stored fat for energy, reducing the frequency and intensity of hunger. Patience here is not just a virtue—it's crucial.

Now, let's talk tactics: staying hydrated is a silver bullet for mitigating hunger. Water doesn't just quench your thirst; it can also fill your stomach and trick your brain into feeling sated. And if plain water bores you to tears, infuse it with some citrus or mint for a refreshing twist.

Diving even deeper, strategic meal timing within your eating window is key. Prioritizing foods rich in fiber, protein, and healthy fats will keep you fuller for longer. It's like building a dam to hold back the hunger tide—construct it well, and you'll stay dry.

Another crucial element is staying busy. An idle mind often leads to an idle stomach. Engage in activities that keep your mind off food. Read that book you've been putting off, take a leisurely walk, or dive into a new hobby. Distraction can be a powerful ally in your battle against cravings.

Speaking of battles, don't arm your cravings with triggers. If scrolling through food blogs or staring at the office candy jar sparks your appetite, change your line of sight. Out of sight truly can be out of mind in these scenarios.

Let's not forget about the power of routine. Establishing a consistent fasting schedule aligns your body's hunger hormones with your eating pattern, gradually easing the intensity of your hunger pangs. Think of it as training your stomach to expect food at certain times, and eventually, it'll stop raising the alarm outside these windows.

Moreover, mindfulness is a potent tool for managing hunger and cravings. Eating mindfully during your allotted times fosters a better relationship with food. Chew slowly, savor every bite, and listen to your body's satiety signals. It's about quality, not just quantity.

An important reminder: Don't be too hard on yourself if you occasionally slip up. Fasting isn't about perfection; it's about persistence and learning from each experience. A misstep can be a valuable lesson in disguise, showing you where your vulnerabilities lie and how you can fortify your strategy.

Support systems shouldn't be underrated. Surrounding yourself with others who understand your fasting lifestyle or joining online communities can provide encouragement and deter you from caving into cravings. Shared journeys are often more manageable, as they say.

Supplements can also play a role. For some, a multivitamin or electrolyte supplement may assist in maintaining energy levels and reducing cravings that stem from nutrient deficiencies. It's like giving your body the right ammunition to fight the hunger battle.

Cognitive behavioral strategies can also be impactful. Identifying the thoughts and behaviors that lead to cravings enables you to address them head-on. Replace a negative habit with a positive one, and soon, the cravings will lose their grip.

Sometimes, the best strategy is sleep. Poor sleep can disrupt hunger hormones and lead to increased appetite. By ensuring you get ample quality sleep, you're setting the stage for more manageable hunger levels during your fasting period.

In conclusion, handling hunger and cravings is a multifaceted endeavor. It's a mix of physical, psychological, and strategic elements. But with the right tools and mindset, you can navigate these waters smoothly. Remember, each day of fasting is a step toward mastering your body's cues and discovering a sense of liberation in your eating habits.

Intermittent fasting isn't about denying yourself the joys of food—it's about rediscovering them in a harmonious balance that supports your health and happiness. So take each hunger pang as a signal to reflect, adjust, and learn. With each fast, you grow stronger, and your control over cravings becomes more resolute. You're not just transforming your eating patterns; you're transforming your life.

Addressing Plateaus and Setbacks

It's the journey through crests and troughs that makes the weight loss experience unique for each individual. Encountering a plateau or experiencing a setback can feel discouraging. Still, it's a normal part of the process, especially while fasting intermittently. Although we've covered various aspects of fasting, right now we'll zero in on what to do when progress stalls, or you find yourself seemingly taking a step back.

Let's talk about plateaus first. They're like that unwelcome guest at your party who just refuses to leave—even when you thought everything was going smoothly. When the scale won't budge, or your clothes don't feel any looser, it's essential not to panic. Our bodies are complex systems, and weight loss isn't linear. Sometimes, they need a moment to recalibrate before the pounds continue to drop.

What about when you're doing everything 'by the book', and suddenly, life throws a curveball that disrupts your well-crafted routine? Maybe it's a stressful period at work, a family emergency, or even holidays that derail your fasting schedule. These instances are setbacks, and while they can be frustrating, they're not the end of your fasting story.

Firstly, remember that resilience is key. Setbacks are temporary, and they bring valuable lessons. Take a moment to reflect on what caused the interruption. Was it a change in routine? Emotional eating? Once you identify the triggers, you can create a strategy for the next time a similar scenario arises. Tweak your approach, plan ahead, or find new coping mechanisms that don't revolve around food.

Secondly, plateaus can sometimes be a sign that your body has adjusted to your current fasting routine, and it may be time to switch things up. Introduce minor changes incrementally: push your fasting window an hour longer, adjust your calorie intake, or add some high-intensity workouts into your week. Keep your body guessing—it's a great way to kick-start the weight loss engine again.

Another aspect to consider is stress and sleep. Are you finding yourself awake at night, worrying about the numbers on the scale? Chronic stress and lack of sleep wreak havoc on your hormones, particularly cortisol, which can promote weight retention. Make sure you're getting enough rest and managing your stress effectively—your body will thank you by functioning optimally.

It's also useful to reassess your eating habits. Are your meals still aligning with your goals? Sometimes we can slowly drift into old eating patterns without realizing it. A piece of cake here, a glass of wine there—it adds up. Make sure that your eating window is filled with nourishing, whole foods that support your fasting journey.

Consulting with a nutritionist or a fasting-friendly healthcare provider can also provide you with personalized solutions. They can help you look at your situation objectively and possibly identify things you may have overlooked. Even the subtlest of changes in your regimen can help break through a weight loss plateau or overcome a setback.

Hydration is another angle to consider. Sometimes we mistake thirst for hunger, leading to unnecessary snacking or overeating. Make sure you're drinking plenty of water throughout your eating and fasting windows. It keeps you full, aids in the metabolic process, and is essential for overall health.

Moreover, don't underestimate the power of a support system. Engaging with a community of like-minded fasters can encourage you when things get tough. Share your struggles, ask for advice, and celebrate the small victories together. Success feels even sweeter when it's shared.

Journaling your journey can be an incredibly insightful tool. Record not just what you eat and when you fast, but also how you feel physically and emotionally. Over time, patterns may emerge that could reveal hidden reasons behind a plateau or setback. Recognizing these patterns empowers you to make informed adjustments.

Remember, weight is not the only measure of success. Sometimes the scale might not move, but you could be losing inches or noticing a change in body composition. Muscle weighs more than fat, so if you're combining fasting with exercise, you might be gaining muscle. Measure your success by how you feel, how your clothes fit, and your overall health, not just by the gravity-pulling numbers.

Finally, perseverance is the ultimate difference-maker. No successful journey lacks challenges; whether you face plateaus or setbacks, staying the course is paramount. Remind yourself why you started fasting—maybe it's for health, longevity, or to feel your best. Keep these motivations at the forefront of your mind to steer you back on the path.

Integrating fasting into your lifestyle is a transformative process, and it's okay to take it one step at a time. A plateau or setback doesn't spell failure; it's an opportunity to learn, grow, and evolve in your fasting practice. You have the power to continue shaping your journey and forging a route that aligns with your life. Let's embrace the ebbs and flows; it's part of the art of fasting and refining our individual paths to wellness.

Conclusion

Integrating Fasting into Your Lifestyle for Lasting Success

If you've journeyed with us through the winding paths and the peaks of insight provided in the preceding chapters, you're standing at a significant threshold. It's the point where knowledge begins to weave seamlessly into the fabric of daily life. The concept of interweaving fasting into the very essence of your lifestyle isn't just the culmination of this discussion—it's the key to unlocking lasting success in your health and wellness journey.

Let's face it: traditional diets often have an expiration date, a time when the energy and motivation wane, and old habits creep back in. However, fasting isn't a fly-by-night diet trend; it's an age-old practice that's backed by modern science and can be tailored to your unique life. And that's the beauty of it—the adaptability and flexibility that fasting offers can help it become a mainstay in your life, not a temporary guest.

Integrating fasting into your life starts with a vision—a vision of you at your healthiest. Picture it: you're radiant, full of energy, free from the yo-yo grip of dieting because you've adopted an approach that's as natural as sleep. Imagine not being bound by the shackles of fad diets, but instead having the freedom to listen to your body's cues and respond in a way that supports your well-being.

To get there, remember that fasting is a personal journey. You can't adopt a one-size-fits-all method. Consider not only your physical health but also your lifestyle, routines, job, family life, and, most importantly, your mental and emotional state. Adjust the intensity and the timing of your fasts to fit your life, not the other way around. Doing so transforms fasting from a regimen to a routine, from a task to a pleasure, from a challenge to a choice.

Addressing the psychological barriers you encountered in Chapter 5, you've learned that embracing fasting is as much about mindset as mechanics. You've built the mental fortitude to see fasting not as deprivation but as replenishment—of health, vigor, and vitality. By recognizing that hunger is not an emergency and cravings are fleeting, you've gained control over the impulses that once swayed your dietary decisions.

Combining the nutritional strategies of Chapter 6, recognize the importance of what you eat, not just when you eat. Refueling your body with nutrient-dense foods post-fast nourishes your body. It cements the gains you've made, fostering a cycle of sustenance that facilitates recovery and prepares you for your next fasting window. This synergy is your secret weapon in making intermittent fasting work harmoniously within your lifestyle.

Let's not forget the physical aspect—fasting and exercise, as explored in Chapter 7. This powerful duo can take your health and fitness to unprecedented levels. By optimizing workout performance around your fasting schedule, you'll find that not only can you sustain a high level of physical activity, but you'll potentially excel at it, thanks to improved metabolic flexibility and energy utilization.

Hormonal harmony is not just a blissful phrase—it's a tangible state you can achieve through fasting, as detailed in Chapter 8. With improved insulin sensitivity and balanced hormones, your body can operate at its finest, turning you into a well-oiled machine that can store energy efficiently and burn fat effectively. These aren't just physiological changes—they are transformative experiences that can redefine how you feel each day.

Women have unique considerations, as discussed in Chapter 9. Embracing these and customizing your fasting strategy to match your body's needs across different stages of life is critical. It respects your body's natural rhythms and helps you to navigate through times of hormonal change with grace and confidence.

In Chapter 10, we delved into managing the social and lifestyle factors that come with a fasting lifestyle. You've learned that being open, planning, and sometimes just being stealthy about your fasting can allow you to enjoy the societal aspects of eating while sticking to your commitments. You can dine out, travel, and celebrate without fasting becoming a hurdle.

Advanced fasting protocols in Chapter 11 showed you how to step up your fasting game, should you choose to. These are not for everyone, but knowing that there is a deeper layer to fasting, like autophagy, gives you something to consider as you grow in your fasting practice.

Finally, Chapter 12 armed you with answers to common questions and strategies to troubleshoot issues that arise. Plateaus might still occur; they're a natural part of any weight loss journey. Yet, now you're equipped with the knowledge and tools to navigate them successfully without throwing in the towel.

Hold onto the fact that fasting is more about rhythm than rigidity. It's about finding your cadence and dancing to the beat of your own drum.

As you move forward, return to the principles outlined in these pages, and adjust as life shifts and changes—it's expected and completely normal.

Lastly, remember the reason you started on this path. You sought something different because you knew something needed to change. Now, with the secret of intermittent fasting unfolding before you, take a moment to appreciate how far you've come. Forge ahead with excitement and curiosity for the endless possibilities that await as you integrate fasting into your lifestyle for lasting success.

The path to understanding how and why traditional diets fail has brought you to the threshold of a new terrain—fasting as a way of life. It's within this journey that you will find not just the answers, but also the lasting success in health and vitality that you've sought after. Fasting isn't just a diet; it's a lifestyle. And as with any meaningful lifestyle change, it's all about weaving new habits into the tapestry of daily life, one thread at a time.

Appendix A
Sample Fasting Schedules and Recipes

You've explored the labyrinth of nutrition and fasted your way through the enigma of weight loss. Now, it's time to put that knowledge into practice. This appendix is your practical guide, leading you towards integrating fasting into your life with ease and enjoyment. Fasting needn't be a solo journey of blandness. Imagine combining effective fasting schedules with delectable recipes suited to your post-fast meals - and we're here to do just that.

Sample Fasting Schedules

Every individual's schedule is unique, so flexibility is key when integrating fasting into your life. Here are a few sample fasting schedules that you can tweak to fit your personal rhythm:

1. **16/8 Method:** Breakfast might be on hiatus with this popular fasting protocol. You fast for 16 hours each day, which includes your sleep time, and eat during an 8-hour window. For example, finishing dinner at 8 PM and eating your next meal at 12 PM is a common approach with the 16/8 method.

2. **5:2 Plan:** With this more flexible option, you're on your regular diet for 5 days of the week, and for 2 non-consecutive days, you limit yourself to 500-600 calories. It's not full fasting, but significantly reduced caloric intake can lead to similar benefits.

3. **Alternate-Day Fasting:** This one's a bit more advanced. You fully fast every other day or limit yourself to about 500 calories on fasting days. The non-fasting days? Eat as you normally would. Plenty of water, herbal teas, or black coffee can help you endure the hunger pangs on fasting days.

4. **One Meal A Day (OMAD):** As its name implies, OMAD involves consuming just one meal a day—preferably a big, nutritious one. That meal should provide your nutrient needs without overindulging. It could be lunch or dinner, depending on your lifestyle.

Whatever method speaks to you, remember – it's not set in stone. Experiment with different patterns and adjust times to find what feels right and is sustainable. It's about finding your personal symphony in the world of fasting.

Nourishing Recipes To Break Your Fast

Let's dive into some recipes that pack a punch with nutrients and flavors, perfect for your eating windows. Remember, breaking your fast should be gentle, starting with something easier on your stomach before you launch into a full meal.

- **Avocado and Berry Salad with Walnuts:** Why not start with a shot of omega-3s, fibers, and antioxidants? Mash half an avocado, toss in a cup of mixed berries, sprinkle with a handful of walnuts, drizzle a bit of balsamic vinegar and you've got a light yet replenishing salad that's perfect for easing out of your fasting period.

- **Quinoa and Roasted Vegetable Bowl:** For the main affair, how about a hearty bowl that combines fluffy quinoa with a variety of roasted vegetables like zucchini, bell peppers, and cherry tomatoes? Drizzle them with olive oil, roast until tender, and mix with cooked quinoa. Add a pinch of sea salt and a squeeze of lemon for an extra zing!

- **Grilled Chicken with Steamed Greens:** Looking for a protein kick? Grill up some chicken seasoned with herbs, and pair it with a side of steamed greens like spinach or kale. This meal is not only savory, but it gives you the necessary protein plus a heap of vitamins and minerals to replenish your body.

Fast-breaking should be an experience that excites your palate and respects your body's needs. Use these recipes as a canvas; feel free to experiment with different herbs, spices, and ingredients to suit your taste buds and nutritional requirements. Who says you can't have your cake – or, in this case, a nourishing meal – and eat it too?

As you flip through these pages, remember: each fast is a step towards a healthier, more vibrant you. Steer clear of the snares of fad diets and sail through your fasting journey with confidence and a sprinkle of culinary creativity. Enjoy each meal, relish in the simplicity of fasting, and let your body thank you in its language of thriving wellness. Bon appétit!

Appendix B
Tracking Progress and Results

o, you've embarked on this intermittent fasting journey, and you're flooding your body with all these amazing benefits. But how do you know it's working? How can you concretely measure the fruits of your tenacity and willpower? Let's talk about tracking progress and results, which isn't just about stepping on a scale. It's cracking the code to your body's responses, understanding the narrative of your health, and celebrating the victories beyond mere pounds and inches.

Setting SMART Goals

Before we dive into the specifics, it's crucial to set goals that are Specific, Measurable, Achievable, Relevant, and Time-bound (SMART). Maybe you're aiming to lose 20 pounds, lower your blood sugar levels, or just feel more energized throughout the day—define your finish line, and let's chart the course to get you there.

Gauging Success Beyond Weight

No doubt weight loss might be a central character in your story, but let's not forget about the supporting cast. Your waist measurement, how those jeans fit, or simply observing a more restful sleep can all be indicators of your success. And remember to note these wins down – if you're feeling better, jot it down. If your focus is sharper, make a note. These qualitative notes will serve as important mile markers on your journey.

Blood Work and Biomarkers

Results also show up in the more clinical aspect—your blood work. Cholesterol levels, blood sugar, blood pressure, and inflammation markers are all tangible results impacted by intermittent fasting. Keep an eye on these figures with regular check-ins with your healthcare provider and watch the narrative of your health evolve.

The Power of Pictures

Let's not underestimate the visual power of before-and-after photos. Snapping a picture every couple of weeks can reveal changes your mirror might be keeping a secret. Sometimes, progress is silent and shy, only showing up in a side-by-side comparison that screams, "Look at how much you've accomplished!"

App-Assisted Accountability

We're living in the golden age of technology, so let's use it to our advantage. There's a plethora of apps dedicated to tracking fasting periods, dietary intake, water consumption, and activity levels. They can lend a hand in staying on track and maintaining the focus required to make intermittent fasting a seamless part of your lifestyle.

Journaling the Journey

Here's where you get to channel your inner writer. Keep a journal documenting your fasting hours, what you're eating during your feeding windows, and any thoughts or feelings that arise. Not only is this therapeutic, but it provides an insightful record of what works for your body—and what doesn't.

The Scale: A Tool, Not a Tyrant

The scale can be useful, but giving it total control over your mood or self-worth isn't the way to go. It's just one data point among many. Focusing too much on your earth-gravity measurement can overshadow other significant successes. Weigh yourself if you like, but maybe limit it to once a week at the same time of day for consistency's sake.

Remember, the proof of your progress isn't solely in how much you weigh or the number you see on the tape measure. It's in the overall enhancement of your quality of life. The reduction of certain medications, the newfound joy in activities that used to tire you, the increased mental clarity—these are the true crowning achievements of your fasting journey. So, let's applaud every step forward, and use these tools as a means to celebrate all facets of your success with intermittent fasting.

One Final Task

Now that you're well on your way to long-lasting, sustainable weight loss and a healthy mindset, you're in the perfect position to hand the baton to the next person. Simply by sharing your honest opinion of this book and a little about your own journey, you'll show new readers where they can finally find the guidance they've been looking for.

IN UNDER 1 MINUTE YOU CAN HELP OTHERS JUST LIKE YOU BY LEAVING A REVIEW

Please use the QR code below to leave your review.

DAVID ALEXANDER

Made in United States
North Haven, CT
25 February 2024

49210912R00075